T0361649

# Face
# in the
# Mirror

JACK EL-HAI

# Face in the Mirror

A SURGEON, A PATIENT, AND THE
REMARKABLE STORY OF THE FIRST
FACE TRANSPLANT AT MAYO CLINIC

MAYO CLINIC PRESS

**Proceeds from the sale of every book benefit important medical research and education at Mayo Clinic.**

To stay informed about Mayo Clinic Press, please subscribe to our free e-newsletter at MCPress.MayoClinic.org or follow us on social media. For bulk sales, contact Mayo Clinic at SpecialSalesMayoBooks@mayo.edu.

**Image Credits** All photographs and illustrations are copyright of Mayo Foundation for Medical Education and Research (MFMER) except for the first photo in the insert, courtesy of Andy Sadness, and the photos on page 15 in the insert, courtesy of Lilly Warborg.

MAYO CLINIC PRESS
200 First St. SW
Rochester, MN 55905

MCPress.MayoClinic.org

ISBN: 979-8-88770-028-1 (hardcover) | 979-8-88770-172-1 (ebook)

Library of Congress Control Number: 2024056645

Library of Congress Cataloging-in-Publication Data is available upon request.

Printed in Canada
First printing: 2025

# Contents

# Author's Note

———

F*ace in the Mirror* is a work of nonfiction. Nothing in it has been fictionalized, and no situations, scenes, or dialogue is invented.

Although Mayo Clinic staff members assisted me in my reporting by suggesting interviewees and giving me access to them, I had independence in choosing my paths of research and following the questions and threads of the story that I believed were most important. I researched the book in three stages. First, I studied the medical literature on the history of facial reconstruction, vascularized composite allotransplantation (VCA, the transplantation of multiple types of tissues from a donor to a patient, often involving a hand or face), and the techniques, risks, and postoperative care of face transplants in particular. Since 2010, that literature has mushroomed, with thousands of articles now in print in medical journals. I then dove into the mass of articles in newspapers, magazines, and online publications about Andy Sandness, the patient whose story is the focus of this book, as well as accounts of the face transplants of other patients.

Next, I began interviewing Andy's lead surgeon, Samir Mardini, and some three dozen surgeons, physicians, therapists, nurses, surgical technologists, photographers, healthcare administrators, social workers, and LifeSource staff involved in his treatment. Starting in 2019, I interviewed Andy many times over four years, in person, by phone, and remotely by video. I also interviewed Andy's family members, including his father, Reed, and wife, Kim, along with other people with roles in his story. Most of these interviews occurred in person at Mayo Clinic or in other places of business, but some took place as video or phone calls. No topics were off-limits in these interviews.

Finally, one of the most time-consuming parts of my research process was to review Andy's voluminous Mayo Clinic medical record—some eighty thousand pages—covering the years 2006 to the present. Andy graciously gave me permission to access this documentation of every aspect of his care in Rochester. Some of the comments of Andy's caregivers included in the book come from this complex documentation of his progress from his gunshot wound to his facial reconstruction to his face transplant.

After I wrote an early draft of the book's manuscript, Andy and Samir Mardini reviewed several drafts of the book's manuscript for accuracy. In my writing, I tried to strike a balance between Andy Sandness's need for privacy and the obligations I always feel to you, the reader, to clearly report on what you need to know to understand the story. Sometimes the balance was tricky to achieve. In the end, though, I can assure you that everything in this book is accurate and true to the experiences of the people involved. This is Andy's story. I hope it resonates with you.

*Chapter 1*

# Momentous

———

Traffic was sparse in downtown Rochester, Minnesota. It was a June Saturday, and even before dawn, the day was gathering the warmth and humidity of early summer. Inside Mayo Clinic Hospital, Saint Marys Campus, the air was cool. A large surgical team had gathered quickly in response to calls and texts asking them to report in for work. A quiet, intense energy hummed in the atmosphere. This was it—the moment they had been training for over the past three years.

Just days earlier, Andy Sandness had traveled alone from his home in Wyoming to Mayo Clinic in Rochester. Standing outside the sprawling brick walls of Saint Marys, he did not know what to expect. Inside the building, he was greeted by Dr. Samir Mardini. The plastic surgeon was waiting for him in a preoperative room. They had known each other for about a decade, since 2006, shortly after Andy had shot himself in the head but survived and was left with a grievously wounded face.

After supervising his patient's prep for surgery, Mardini gave Andy a final consent form to sign. Andy affirmed that he fully understood the risks of the extraordinarily complex surgical procedure he was about to undergo—a face transplant, never before undertaken at Mayo Clinic. He signed without hesitation and, it seemed to Mardini, with evident composure. "Is this something you're sure you want to do?" Mardini asked a final time. "If so, we're ready to go."

Andy replied, "Yes, I'm ready." Over the past few years, they had spoken many times about what was coming. Now there was nothing more to say. Andy and Mardini hugged. Their emotions ran high, but they shared an inner calm. After working hard to reach this stage, both men felt ready for the hard work ahead of them.

As Andy waited to enter the operating room, he said a little prayer. He prayed for himself, for Mardini, for the Mayo Clinic team, and for the family of the brain-dead young man, nearby in the same hospital, whose face soon would become Andy's own.

Mardini walked alongside him as staff members pushed him in a wheelchair toward the operating suite. Wanting to lighten the mood, the surgeon, who would use his entire medical training in this surgery, pulled out his phone and showed Andy a video of his own two small children playing. Together, they entered the operating room where Andy's transplant would take place. In the adjoining suite, the preparation of the donor was beginning. Mardini turned to his patient. "We're looking forward to seeing you with a new face," he said.

Years later, Andy remembers climbing onto the operating table and beseeching the nurse, "Please don't let anything bad happen to me."

"Don't you worry about that," she replied.

She grasped his hand as Andy drifted into a chemically induced sleep. He would not fully awaken for ten days. Watching Andy, the nurse thought, "Wow, we're here. Andy's here. We know this is the right thing to do." All involved in the surgery knew their role in what was to follow. Of the hundreds of procedural steps ahead, each one had been thought out and rehearsed many times.

∽

On the way to this momentous day in his life, Andy had already experienced the gamut of human emotions, from deep despair to soaring hope. Nearly a decade had passed since he had attempted to take his own life. His great regret for doing so did not erase the depression that had led up to the attempt. And although he was glad to be alive, he was left with a disfigurement that was painfully obvious to him and the rest of the world. More than anything, Andy wanted to look and feel ordinary. He wanted to walk into a room and talk to people without anyone scrutinizing his face or asking him awkward questions. He wanted to cast away the clumsy prosthetic nose that required daily cleaning with a toothbrush. He wanted to eat like he used to. He wanted to swim. He wanted to kiss.

When Andy first learned of the possibility of a face transplant, his response had been an enthusiastic endorsement of the idea. But Mardini had urged him to slow down and consider all that could happen, including the possibility of failure.

At times, the complexity and high stakes of the surgery had made Andy waver. Once, after a three-day stay at Mayo Clinic, pondering all the information he had been presented about the procedure, he decided he did not want to go through with it. The risk was too great, and he felt overwhelmed by the magnitude of it all. The operation would demand too much of him, and a bad outcome would be disastrous. If Mardini could not successfully graft the extensive network of new tissue onto Andy's skull, Andy might be left with a large, gaping hole in his face. And if Andy's body rejected the new tissue, he could expect endless dangers and complications. Sensing Andy's uncertainty, Andy's father pulled him aside and asked if he really wanted to walk away from the possible future he yearned for.

At his next evaluation, Andy had felt more upbeat. He considered himself a good candidate for the procedure: He had the support of his family and was in excellent health except for his facial disfigurement. His tally of the pros and cons of undergoing the surgery made clear what the operation might allow him to do that he could not do now. He might recover full functioning of his lips, teeth, and nose, and his appearance could greatly improve.

Or perhaps not. That was the uncertainty. The results of a face transplant varied wildly among the small number of people—just over three dozen—who had undergone the procedure. Afterward, he might not be able to smile, close his lips, or speak intelligibly. He might continue to look disfigured, just in a different way.

To make the surgery a success, both before and after the procedure, Andy would have to maintain a physically and mentally healthy life, show resilience, overcome daunting obstacles, and, above all, develop optimism. Regardless of the efforts of the people whose labors were set to synchronize in a vast medical symphony, only Andy could give himself what he needed to live a fulfilled and happy life. He had decided to move ahead with preparing for the transplant.

On this day, Saturday, June 11, 2016, Andy was on the brink of a new life. He felt ready. The massive surgical team assembled to treat him was also ready.

Next door was the other young man, the donor, whose organs were being kept alive by medical machines.

The procedure began. Soon there would be no way to turn back. In total, about fifty doctors, nurses, and other Mayo staff prepared to spend the next fifty-six hours giving Andy a new face, his second chance. Would the vastly complex surgery transform Andy's life the way he hoped?

# Chapter 2

# "My Son Is Dead"

———

A ndy had always been a determined kid, even as an infant. Following his birth in 1985 in Custer, South Dakota, he was hospitalized for failure to thrive at the age of three months. Once doctors discovered he had several food allergies, however, he was treated, and he fully recovered.

When he was three or four, living with his family in Moorcroft, Wyoming (population then 772), he remembers riding around on his bicycle—one of his first times riding without training wheels. Behind him he towed his old tricycle with the front wheel and steering column removed. It must have looked strange, a boy leaning into his pedals to propel a mismatched and spinning combination of wheels and frames and spokes. He rode in countless circles. It winded him, and it satisfied his need to feel busy and active.

Like most families, Andy's has its own story of love and loss. Andy has never known his biological father, who left Andy's mother, Rhonda, and his older sister, Rhiannon, when Andy was only a baby. "I don't even know if he's still alive," Andy says. "I don't really care." He looks to Reed Sandness, his stepfather, as his true father, the one who raised him.

Andy vividly remembers his introduction to his younger brother, Ronald. Reed had told him to get ready for a day of fishing. They hopped into the family van and drove for a half hour to the town of Sundance, where they stopped in the parking lot of a hospital. "This isn't the lake," Andy thought. When he got out of the van, looked at the roof of the vehicle, and saw no fishing poles strapped on, he felt confused.

They weren't really going fishing, Reed acknowledged. "Your mom is having a baby," he said. Andy, three years old, didn't know what to expect when they walked into his mother's room. There was Rhonda with a tiny baby boy in her arms. "It's your brother," she told Andy. Incredulous, Andy held the new family member, Ronald. He felt excited and proud, and vowed to be the best big brother he could be.

Two years after Ronald's birth, the family moved from Moorcroft to Upton, Wyoming. Their new place had a swing set, a tree fort, and seventeen acres for Andy and Ronald to explore. Andy recalls getting up at sunrise, excited to play outside. He and Ronald played outdoors together all summer, and every childhood summer thereafter, with no supervision. They came inside mainly to eat and sleep. The boys rarely went into town; they had only each other for company.

Andy took his role as Ronald's big brother seriously. When they found a wasp nest hidden inside an old dump truck, Ronald offered to get rid of it. Andy would not allow this. He was the older brother, he had lived longer, Andy told Ronald. If anybody was going to die, it was going to be Andy. He knocked the nest off the truck, and as it hit the ground the boys took off running. They were back playing inside the cab of that dump truck the next day. And when they weren't at the dump truck, Andy was pushing

Ronald for hours in a Power Wheels car with a dead battery. The boys broke windows and started minor fires. Ronald was Andy's main playmate and best friend.

The Sandness family raised chickens, geese, ducks, pheasants, and puppies. Andy and Ronald, meanwhile, became enamored with dirt biking. They shared a bike and rode it around everywhere.

Andy's father, Reed, was away working on a railroad most of the time, but Andy remembers fishing with him and spending time together outdoors, sometimes near Reed's hometown of Mitchell, South Dakota, and sometimes at a reservoir in the low hills of northeastern Wyoming. They would rise early to fish. "We never caught anything, but we'd always go out and always tried," Andy says.

Beyond fishing, the father and son were not frequent companions when Andy was young. Reed drank. "He was always rough around the edges," Andy says. "I think it's the way he was raised. He didn't know any better when he raised us." Reed had not been close to his own father, and fatherhood at a distance seemed almost normal in the Sandness family. Reed coped by being strict, just as his father had been. Andy remembers getting punished by Reed for using foul language in the public library and for other juvenile infractions.

A tough work ethic is one thing Andy is glad to have received from his father. "You've got to feed the chickens, clean the chicken coop, do all this stuff," Andy says. "That's how he was raised, and that's how he raised us."

Sometimes Rhonda relied on Andy for responsibilities beyond his years. When Andy was about ten, she asked him to build steps for the front porch of the family home. Using a circular saw, he cut pieces of wood and mounted them in the semblance of a staircase. "They were terrible, but they worked," Andy says. Rhonda praised him for his effort. "I tried to be a handyman for her, and she just loved that."

During Andy's middle school years, his parents separated for a time. Reed moved out, and Rhonda remained in the family house with the kids. She struggled financially but was protective of her children. Andy's memories of those middle school years are sketchy, and he recalls little about his parents' time apart, aside from certain details: "We didn't have money for heat. We ended up moving in with one of my mom's friends, and there were seven of us living in a two- or three-bedroom trailer house. Thank God they took us in," he says.

Andy didn't know anyone who had survived a rougher upbringing than his mother, a native of West Virginia. When she was very young, her brother and mother had died in quick succession. Rhonda became an expert at handling death and tending to graves. She mowed, pulled weeds, and planted flowers at the grave sites of people she knew. Rhonda had other bad memories from West Virginia, dark events she was reluctant to discuss. Her childhood experiences made her never want to return there to live. But she would sometimes go back to visit. Minus Reed, the family took many road trips there, on one occasion making it from Wyoming to West Virginia in twenty-four hours with Andy squabbling with Rhiannon and Ronald the whole way there.

When Andy was around twelve, Ronald broke his arm. "That just sucked for him," Andy says, "because it was his right arm that got broken and he couldn't push the [dirt bike's] throttle."

A broken arm is a common childhood injury, but worse befell a neighbor boy Andy got to know. Robert White was seven years older than Andy. When Andy was in the fifth grade and Robert a high school senior, Robert died in a car wreck. Andy still remembers the details: "He went off in the ditch, and then he didn't overcorrect. It was just a huge embankment. He had his buddy with him. Somehow Robert died but his friend didn't. . . . He was such a good dude." Andy glimpsed then that the world was a risky place, and that commonplace activities could easily turn into tragedy.

At school, Andy played basketball. One day during seventh grade Andy was playing basketball and wandered off into the locker room, feeling dazed. He didn't know what was happening or what he was doing there. The coach sat Andy out for the rest of the game and talked with Andy's mom that night about the incident. Andy soon came down with mononucleosis-like symptoms that kept him out of school for three months. He believes he spent most of those months playing on his Nintendo 64 and trying to keep up with his schoolwork, but he remembers little of that time. "I have a really good memory, and that's the one time that I really don't have any memories"of, he says.

Other parts of Andy's life felt haphazard and humiliating at times. He was bullied at school by classmates. With money tight, he sometimes called Reed to ask for cash for dog food and the baseball cards he felt guilty for collecting.

Deeper troubles happened as well. At age thirteen, he managed to fend off and escape from a friend's father, a man later convicted as a pedophile, who tried to sexually assault him. The incident left Andy in emotional upheaval. He told Rhonda what had happened, and she arranged for him to meet with a therapist.

When Andy's parents reunited for a time, the family settled in the Wyoming town of Newcastle, which Andy still considers his hometown. Although bigger than Moorcroft and Upton, Newcastle was still a small community, with 3,400 people. But it seemed enormous to Andy—in his initial years there, the town had a bowling alley, a skating rink, and a water park. Andy rode his bicycle everywhere, and he felt free.

Before too long, though, Newcastle's kid-friendly amenities dwindled away, and suddenly there was not much for Andy to do. During the summers he played youth baseball, "and I sucked at it," he says. It was something to do, but his teams were never any good.

Intolerable from Andy's perspective were the public fights between his parents. Once when Andy was playing football with friends, Reed and Rhonda chased each other around a parking lot in their vehicles, in full view of everyone. Driving a Toyota 4Runner, Rhonda plowed into Reed and his Volkswagen van. "We could see this," Andy remembers. "Everyone could see it." He felt embarrassed, and the other kids teased him about it for months.

Feeling like he didn't fit in, Andy decided to change his image. Before high school, he had been a better-than-average student. Now he rebelled. Like many young people in the area, he spent nights and weekends smoking weed and drinking. Andy smoked and drank more than most of his friends. He was often grounded at home by his parents. "All the time," Andy says. But that did not stop him from holding down odd jobs during high school to earn money. If he wanted to have a car, he needed to have auto insurance; working would pay for that and other bills. Andy believed college was not in his future. "I just partied too much back then," he said.

After finishing high school, Andy went into training with True Oil Company in Vernal, Utah—a small city tucked into the northeastern corner of the state and about eight hours from Newcastle. An accident on the job resulted in a scar on the left side of his face. After a wrenching breakup with a girlfriend around age nineteen, Andy became depressed.

Reed and Rhonda at last divorced in 2005. It was an acrimonious split that Andy tried to stay out of but could not. Andy's sister, Rhiannon, had since moved to West Virginia and was working as a pharmacy assistant, but Ronald remained in Newcastle. Reed and Rhonda placed Andy and Ronald in the middle of endless conflict, involving fights, accusations, and emotional and mental manipulation. "I just went into a super depression," he says of this time in his life. This despondency hung over him for the next year.

∼

By 2006, Andy, now twenty-one, was working full-time as an electrician apprentice at Statewide Electric in Casper, Wyoming. He stayed with his mother in Newcastle on weekends. People who knew Andy saw him as well-liked, kind, and friendly, but also believed he was drinking more heavily than in the past. Few knew he was consuming at least a fifth of hard alcohol daily. He presented a positive picture to Rhonda, however, lying to her by saying he was avoiding smoking pot and refraining from other drugs.

Three days before Christmas in 2006, Andy spent the evening with Reed. They had recently been getting along well, and Andy felt he had mostly healed from his parents' marital conflicts. Now things were better between father and son.

The next night, Rhonda gave Andy a bottle of liquor for him to share with friends. He took it to a raucous party with dozens of other guests. They were all drinking, and so was Andy, heavily. When Rhonda came home in the early hours of the morning of December 24 after bartending, Andy became violently upset. They argued. Andy later said he picked a fight with her. "I started yelling and screaming," he remembers, although he says he never would have tried to physically hurt her.

Unable to explain his despondency, he tried to push her away, to build a wall between her worry and his despair. He could not explain his depression to anyone, not his father, his brother, his sister, or his friends. Intoxicated and agitated, he had reached the bottom of a deep depressive pit. "I just gave up on life right then and there."

Angrily, he stormed upstairs and into his bedroom. He smashed everything he could reach: a mounted deer head he cherished, a TV screen, a picture of Al Pacino as Scarface on the wall. Rhonda retreated to her bedroom. Andy's rage continued, and at about 3:00 a.m., his spinning mind suddenly stopped to focus on the 7mm rifle he knew was in his mother's bedroom closet. He had thought about suicide in the past but never attempted it. Like most people in his community, Andy owned and used firearms for hunting. Weeks earlier he had stored them at a friend's house because he feared he would use them to harm himself, but he had since brought them back home. The thought of killing himself arose when he was angry or sad and frustrated at his inability to express himself. At such times, the idea "I'd be better off dead" rose in his mind.

Now, an impulse seized him. Andy burst into his mother's room shouting "I hate you!" Then he went for the closet. (Rhonda later said she did not know the rifle was there.) He grabbed the gun and returned to his own room. "I put a bullet in the chamber, and I'm crying and sobbing," he said.

The way he saw things, he either had to get treatment for his alcohol dependency or kill himself. In his distress, those were the only two choices he could imagine. On the spot, he made an irrational choice. He felt so angry at the world that he stopped caring about his life. He wanted to get out. "I remember looking down and thinking, 'Oh, fuck it,'" he says. He sat on the bed and set the stock of the rifle between his legs and the barrel of the rifle against his chin. He squeezed the trigger.

The world shook. His mother had followed Andy into his bedroom and saw the rifle fire. Andy's body rose from the bed and into the air before falling back down. She screamed in terror and found a phone. She told the 911 dispatcher, "My son is dead—he just shot himself."

But Andy was not dead. After the blast, he remained semiconscious, and the thought drifted to him that he had made an enormous mistake. He curled up on his bed and started screaming and crying. Then he dropped to the floor. He did not know how long he remained in this position or where his mother was.

The bullet had shot away his nose, his jaw, and most of his teeth. Andy's mouth, or what was left of it, was unrecognizable.

His eyes were seriously damaged. His first clear memory was of a childhood friend named Ryan Kerns standing above him. Kerns was a Newcastle police officer at the time.

"Hey, man, are you all right?" was all Kerns could think to say, although it must have been clear that Andy was far from well. Andy, still crying, tried to tell Kerns he was in bad shape. He tried to say, "I don't want to die, Ryan. Don't let me die." But he could not speak the words, or any words at all.

Kerns cradled Andy in his arms and tried to calm him. After a stretch of minutes that Andy could not measure, an ambulance arrived. Emergency medical technicians placed him on a gurney. When they brought him downstairs, he sensed that his mother was waiting in the living room. Andy wanted to talk to her, to apologize to her. He did not understand the seriousness of his condition. He only felt he had let his mother down, along with his whole family.

The EMTs were busy stanching his bleeding and covering his wound. They knew there was no time to waste and rushed him to the front door. They needed to get him to a hospital immediately. "I remember picking my head up and then looking at my mom and trying to say 'I'm sorry,'" he says, "and then they took me into the ambulance."

He became combative. The EMTs wanted to cut off his coat, which he resisted because he had bought it only recently. He struggled and pleaded with them to free his arms, believing he could remove the coat himself without them slicing it. The rifle shot had left Andy confused, frightened, remorseful, and unaware of his injuries.

On arrival at the eighteen-bed Weston County hospital in Newcastle, he underwent a computed tomography (CT) scan that, unexpectedly, showed no injuries to his brain. The bullet had committed vicious damage along its path, but it had missed the brain. Reed, who had received a phone call telling him that Andy shot himself and probably would not survive, rushed to the hospital. He entered his son's room and saw Andy with his entire head wrapped in bandages. The Newcastle physicians, recognizing that Andy's injuries were beyond their capabilities, were preparing him for transfer to a larger regional hospital in Rapid City, South Dakota, seventy-eight miles from Newcastle.

Upon arrival in Rapid City, Andy was still responsive to the voices of the hospital staff and could follow simple instructions. They also could see he needed more intensive emergency care than they could provide, and Andy spent only a couple of hours there. Andy received two units of red blood cells, a catheter to drain his urine, and a tetanus booster vaccine. The hospital staff packed and carefully rewrapped Andy's torn face. They moved Andy—now intubated so that he could breathe and in an induced coma—onto a waiting air ambulance with instructions to fly him over the state line into Minnesota.

Andy arrived on Christmas Eve night at the Emergency Department of Saint Marys, part of the Mayo Clinic medical campus in Rochester, Minnesota. The head of the Division of Trauma Surgery, Scott Zietlow, was on call that night.

Over the years, Zietlow had seen others come in with gunshot wounds like Andy's. Many did not survive, and many did not even make it alive to a hospital. None of the injuries was exactly the same as any of the others, but they all followed a similar pattern: loss of much of the lower and upper jaw and severe damage to the lower part of the face. In many of these cases, because of the angle at which the firearm was placed against the chin, a reflexive tilt of the head from the impact caused the shot to miss the patient's brain. Even if life was tenuously preserved, the outcome was a tremendous amount of facial injury and damage. The loss of blood, risk of infection, and threat of complications were high. If Andy was to be like others before him, he might well die after arriving at the hospital.

The Emergency Department staff unwrapped the bandages and layers of dressing underneath to examine Andy's face, and then covered him with warm blankets. Their first task was to give him a way to breathe reliably. An oral endotracheal tube was keeping his airway open, but one staff member had to hold it in place continuously because of the width of Andy's facial wound.

Within thirty minutes of his arrival at Mayo, Andy was wheeled into an operating room to have a tracheostomy tube inserted a few centimeters above the collarbones. The tracheostomy would provide a more secure breathing line, bypassing Andy's mouth and nose to open a breathing hole in his trachea. Andy, although still unconscious, was sometimes reflexively agitated and a serious and immediate danger to himself. The staff placed him in cloth limb restraints.

Once Andy's access to air had been ensured, he needed blood, and lots of it. A new CT scan confirmed that his brain was uninjured. It also showed that the self-inflicted gunshot had caused extensive damage to the center of his face, including fragmentation of his upper and lower jaws, mouth, nose, and sinuses. Fortunately, the tongue was intact; the concussive effect of the rifle blast may have knocked it back out of the path of the bullet. In addition, his eye orbital bones and cheekbones were fractured. He suffered choroidal ruptures—breaks in the tissue in the middle layer of the walls of both eyes—as well as hemorrhaging in the left eye. Both eyes were swollen shut. The scan revealed bullet fragments in the middle portion of his face plus pockets of air and fluid. It seemed incredible that Andy's brain had not suffered injuries. Another favorable sign: examination showed his vision was intact, although damaged.

Zietlow believed, considering the seriousness of Andy's wounds and his reliance on the full support of a ventilator, that Andy was doing reasonably well. Checking Andy's wounds, he found no active bleeding. His immediate plan for Andy, after ensuring adequate pain control, sedation, and antibiotic administration, was to take a magnetic resonance imaging (MRI) scan of the spine to ensure there was no damage to bones or ligaments. Next, and soon, should come an operation for an open gastrostomy in the abdomen, which would allow the placement of a feeding tube. "There was no way he was going to be eating and drinking, at least in the foreseeable future, with the injuries he had," Zietlow said, "and you have to get him nutrition to heal and to live."

Andy's gastrostomy was scheduled for December 26. While in the operating room, Mayo's facial trauma team would also examine Andy and determine additional treatment. Zietlow obtained consent for the next day's surgery by phone from Rhonda, who, with her friend Kim Fulton and the family's chihuahua, was driving from Newcastle, Wyoming, to Rochester, nine and a half hours away.

Ten years later, when asked for an opinion on Andy's case, Zietlow remembered his patient well. His experience with Andy on Christmas Eve in 2006 was impossible to forget, and Zietlow still clearly recalled details of Andy's arrival. He said he routinely remembers his patients who die during their treatment, but other patients linger in his mind as well. Andy lives in Zietlow's memory because of the devastating injury he'd suffered, the management of which was difficult, involving details and techniques Zietlow continues to pass on to the next generation of surgeons at Mayo.

Despite that high level of care, Andy would need to stay in the intensive care unit (ICU) for a long time.

∽

Andy had wild dreams during his first days in the hospital. In one, he felt desperately worried about his backpack—had he lost it?

Where was it? This dream flowed into another about football. On Christmas Eve, he had planned to watch an NFL game with his friend Kevin, a matchup between the Denver Broncos and the Cincinnati Bengals. "I was dreaming that I ran out on the field and got tackled by Al Wilson, the [Broncos] linebacker, and he put me in the hospital," Andy remembered.

Sedated and grievously wounded, Andy soon grew aware that someone was holding his hand. When he opened his eyes in his hospital room, his mother's face hovered close, with that of his sister, Rhiannon, nearby. Rhonda arrived in Rochester on December 28, and her drive to Rochester, navigated without cellphones or GPS guidance during severe wintry weather, had not been easy. Rhonda's expression, a look Andy will never forget, showed deep pain.

Feeding and breathing tubes coiled into Andy's body. He wanted to speak to his mother, but his injuries made it impossible. Someone brought him a pen and pad of paper. Hurriedly he scrawled, "I'm sorry." Upon reading the message, Rhonda told him she loved him and that it was all right. She seemed to understand his pain and his regret, feelings that had been urgently pressing in upon him, consciously and in dreams, since the moment he pulled the trigger of the rifle.

But it was not all right, for Andy or for Rhonda. His mother's words of understanding did not soothe Andy, whose emotions—despite the sedatives and other medicine coursing through his body—were in turmoil. Even worse than the strange sensations he felt on his damaged face were the agony and guilt he felt for what he had done to the people he loved. Nothing his mother could say would numb him to that pain.

In the days before Rhonda's arrival, Zietlow, after consulting with Mayo Clinic plastic surgeon Samir Mardini, made initial surgical efforts to clean up Andy's face, using suction and sponges to remove loose debris from the gunshot wound. Andy's lower jawbone was nearly all gone, along with most of the upper jaw. He no longer had a nose. Zietlow picked out loose bone chips and cut away damaged tissue. He closed the wounds at the edges of the injured area and packed the open cavity of the face and sinuses when he was done.

A new doctor, critical care surgeon Mark Sawyer, now started managing Andy's treatment in the surgical intensive care unit. Despite the appearance of Andy's horrific wounds, Sawyer expected his patient to survive. Aware that the records arriving with Andy documented his history of alcohol consumption, Sawyer directed the staff to keep watch for symptoms of withdrawal.

Sawyer also worried about the effect of the grievous injuries on Andy's evident depression. He kept Andy sedated for most of the week, gradually lessening the sedation over time. Andy occasionally showed signs of consciousness but remained mostly unconscious and dependent on a ventilator to take his breaths.

That first week was not without challenges. There was a moment when Andy's arms and legs began shaking involuntarily, followed by more quaking in short bursts. A resident observed two episodes of jerky movements of the arms that lasted twenty to thirty seconds. Increased sedation halted the movements, which, to everyone's relief, did not return. Andy's physicians suspected the cause was paroxysmal autonomic phenomena, a movement disorder that sometimes accompanies trauma.

An unrelated problem soon arose: Andy clawed at his feeding and respiration tubes, catheter, and facial bandages even while sedated. The staff continued tying his arms down with cloth restraints. When the staff explained why the restraints were needed, Andy nodded in apparent understanding. However, no one was sure how much Andy was comprehending or remembering. His agitation sometimes required additional sedation, such as when his facial dressings needed changing.

Several times, Andy surprised Sawyer and the other medical staff by giving a thumbs-up sign. In contrast to his otherwise apparent lack of awareness, Andy's gesture appeared to give a different message. "He seemed like he'd gotten a second chance, and he knew it," said Sawyer, who had anticipated that his patient would be less aware. By the end of Sawyer's week on duty, Andy was alert at times, looking around, and making purposeful movements with his hands. "Patient is beginning to wake up," Sawyer noted. "We will continue to minimize his sedation and see how he does off ventilator support for the next 24 hours."

By the first days of 2007, Andy was often alert—although painkillers continued to dull his awareness. He was able to respond to questions by nodding and writing. Luckily, his facial wounds were free of infection.

Andy's eyes had been injured by the gunshot blast but were still intact. His vision in his right eye was 20/30 after the gunshot wound, but the left had much worse perception. He sometimes had to wear a patch over the left eye at the hospital to help himself see clearly with the right eye. Fortunately, both eyes could move freely. The closure of his facial wounds restricted the use of his right eyelid, contributing to the risks to his cornea. Doctors treated Andy with ointment on both eyes while monitoring their healing.

By January 2, Andy was able to have something resembling a conversation with psychiatrist James Rundell, though Andy occasionally nodded off during their encounters. Nodding or shaking his head, Andy acknowledged that he had attempted suicide and that he had wanted to die when he shot himself. Now, he insisted, he wanted to live. Andy "actually held out his hand for me to shake it when I asked him if he wanted to live," Rundell wrote in Andy's medical record. The staff should not worry that he would again try to take his own life, Andy asserted through gestures and head movements. He denied having hallucinations, delusions, illusions, or obsessive ideas. Andy was able to communicate that he felt no significant pain but did not know where he was. "He seemed surprised to hear he was at Mayo Clinic in Rochester, Minnesota," Rundell observed.

Andy consented to his mother making medical decisions for him for now. He still lacked the mental clarity necessary to make his own choices, but Rundell thought Andy might eventually need encouragement to take a more active role in his medical care.

After his first couple of weeks in the hospital, Andy was sometimes able to sit in a chair. A social worker observed that although he could not speak, Andy appeared upbeat. In cases like Andy's, Mayo psychiatrists and psychologists typically recommend concealing serious facial injuries from patients until they express the wish to see them. Andy had not seen his injuries yet, nor shown an interest in doing so.

Gently, as he grew more consistently alert, Andy's physical therapy began. His physical therapist presented modest goals for his recovery. Before his discharge from the hospital, she hoped Andy would be able to safely move by himself from his bed to a chair and vice versa, and she wanted him to be able to stand on his own. The therapist started a regimen of five to nine treatment sessions per week.

Although Andy still felt unsteady on his feet, he quickly began to exceed his therapist's goals. While Rhiannon was visiting, he took short walks around the ICU with her—around his room, a few steps in the hallway, and back to his bed. Each walk amounted to fifty or seventy-five feet.

On one of these strolls, Andy caught sight of a reflection of his bandaged face in a window. The image haunted him. "I'm never going out of this room," he told himself in despair. "I don't want to leave. I don't ever want to see myself like that."

Reliance on others for routine needs also bothered him. He resisted using the bedpan. On one occasion early on, when nature called, he attracted a nurse's attention and pointed to the bathroom in his room. The nurse said he was not yet allowed to use it. He scribbled on a pad, "I can walk over there." The nurse did not relent, and Andy used the bedpan unhappily. It was the last time. From then on, he was determined to totter over to the bathroom every time he needed to use the toilet. Using the bedpan was embarrassing to him, "because all the nurses are looking at you, watching you. I'm a private person," he later said.

But he grew to depend on the Saint Marys ICU staff. These weeks were a sad time for Andy. Anxious over his future, Andy occupied a dark hospital room with dimmed lights because of his sensitivity to glare. Mirrors were covered to avoid distressing him. The staff worked hard to improve his outlook and keep him moving.

With Andy not yet seeing his face, however, his doctors and nurses were uncertain how much he understood about the damage his self-inflicted gunshot had caused. A physician observed that he was expressing a desire to eat and drink normally, "which indicates that the patient is completely unaware of the extent of his injuries."

During these early weeks of his treatment, Andy officially met the Mayo Clinic plastic surgeon who had been on call when Andy was admitted to Saint Marys, who had been consulted on his surgery of December 26, and who would be responsible for Andy's facial reconstruction. The surgeon introduced himself as Samir Mardini. Thirty-six and with a tall, slender build, Mardini had a measured, gentle way of speaking, a high forehead, and kind, dark eyes. He looked at Andy when he talked to him. Andy was struck by the surgeon's calm demeanor and his ability to quickly grasp Andy's worries and needs. Neither of them realized how much their lives would intertwine in the years to come.

Together, Mardini and Sawyer devised a plan for Andy's early facial reconstruction. Even though Andy's ability to pay for medical care was not yet established one way or the other, Mardini assured Andy that he would receive the best treatment Mayo Clinic could offer. "I just need you to be strong and patient," he added. As Andy later remembered, his mom told him, "Don't worry, Andy. They'll fix you up. They're going to fix you up."

# Chapter 3

# Reconstruction

————

S amir Mardini had been hired onto the Mayo Clinic staff less than three months earlier, on October 2, 2006. Up to that point, Mardini's life had followed a very different path than Andy's had.

Born in 1970, in Little Rock, Arkansas, Mardini grew up in a tightly knit Lebanese family. His father, a pediatric cardiologist, had come from Lebanon with his wife to do his residency in Little Rock. Mardini described his father as an old-school practitioner for whom "work [was] really everything." His mother, an interior designer by profession, was a strong and caring woman who prioritized her family and her children. Two years after Mardini was born, another son followed.

After moves to Richmond, Virginia, and Baltimore, where the elder Mardini completed a fellowship at Johns Hopkins University, the family returned to Lebanon in 1974. In Beirut, Mardini's father opened the nation's sole pediatric cardiology clinic. Then civil war erupted. Mardini was young, but he later recalled the turmoil and threat of danger on the streets. In one instance, he and his brother were in a car stuck in a traffic jam when trouble was brewing in the vicinity. Suddenly his father appeared in another car, grabbed his sons, and whisked them away to safety.

Anxious to remove his family from a war zone, Mardini's father took a position at another hospital in the Middle East. The family lived in an American compound, although the boys studied in schools with local children. The elder Mardini's desire had been to return to Lebanon, but this proved untenable. Several times Samir and his brother prepared to transfer to a school in Lebanon, but the dangerous situation in the country always led their father to halt their relocation plans.

At about age ten, Mardini had the opportunity to watch one of his father's colleagues perform an open-heart surgery to repair a defective valve in a young patient's heart. The experience changed his life. "I remember thinking, 'Look at this heart. It's tiny, and it's pumping. How does this thing keep on pumping all the time?'" he said, still with a hint of wonderment in his voice. Back then he had wondered what the surgeon was thinking and experiencing. "What an incredible privilege it is to be in someone's chest and working on one of the most valuable organs. I remember thinking those things, even at ten years old." The ten-year-old Mardini imagined that becoming a surgeon was like taking a journey into an unknown land and returning there fifty or a hundred times until he could see the path clearly and the landscape became familiar.

Surgery's deliberate step-by-step processes intrigued the young boy. "All of it was fascinating: how you can go in and cut up and fix [things]," he said. From then on, he wanted to be a surgeon. Initially he planned to become a pediatric cardiac surgeon, because he believed it would never grow dull. Later, Mardini's wife, Rawan, would describe his fascination with medicine—along with his professional courage and calmness—as coming from his father, and his caring and positive attitude from his mother.

In 1984, the family relocated back to the United States and established their home in the Washington, D.C., area. Now fourteen years old and attending American schools, Mardini entered a period of transition. He felt he didn't fit in at school. He wanted to make friends, but it was a new place, and he felt some cultural differences from his fellow students. The transition to an American high school from a Middle Eastern all-boys educational system was difficult.

Yet, despite the adolescent awkwardness he felt, "good things came out of it," he said. "You're in tune with what others are thinking. You're conscious of every small action you take. You're trying to please others." Those optimistic qualities propelled the young man to prove himself, and to become highly ranked in the opinion of others. The same qualities would later contribute to his sympathetic bedside manner. In high school, Mardini took vocational tests that suggested he would do well in business, but he was bent on a medical career, and those test results pushed him to take charge of his future.

He went on to major in biology at George Washington University, then enrolled in medical school at the Medical College of Virginia. In 1995, after four years of medical school, he was thrilled to match into the general surgical residency at Georgetown University in Washington, D.C. He considered it a dream residency because it was both a top-notch program and located near his family's home in northern Virginia. From the start of his time at Georgetown, Mardini was learning from academic giants in the field, and he loved it. In his classmates and teachers, he found positivity and support. In every year of medical school, he supplemented his surgical training with research. He was thrilled to be moving along his chosen path.

As a surgical resident, Mardini was now operating on patients with his mentors, including the residency program director, Russell Nauta, a figure larger than life who was known for his big heart and sly humor. Nauta had graduated from Harvard and taken a position at Georgetown University. He brought with him an intensity and discipline that translated to all the residents he trained. As Mardini remembers him, Nauta asked a lot and he gave a lot.

Without today's limitations on the length of a resident's workweek, Mardini was typically on call every other day. He might arrive at the hospital on a Monday morning and work through Tuesday evening, go home to sleep, return Wednesday morning and work into the night on Thursday, again sleep at home, and work all day Friday. Then Mardini would be on call through the weekend. The cycle began again the following Monday morning. This exhausting schedule made it hard for Mardini to maintain much of a social life, but that was not a concern for him as he focused on strengthening his surgical skills and increasing his familiarity with surgical patient care.

During his residency, Mardini spent a few months at D.C. General Hospital, a large and hectic trauma center (now closed), which further helped form him as a surgeon. There he took charge of emergency room patients who had suffered gunshot wounds and other serious injuries and who needed immediate cardiac help. He regularly spent consecutive days and nights running between patients in the trauma bay, working to stop massive bleeding, making critical decisions, and sending patients to emergency surgery. These experiences changed his perspective on medicine. Saving lives was thrilling, and it boosted his confidence. "The intense adrenaline and the emotional reward are magnificent," he said.

In his third year of residency, Mardini reached a turning point in his years-long pursuit of a career in pediatric cardiac surgery. Nauta had already arranged interviews for Mardini at Harvard University's Brigham and Women's Hospital to study in the pediatric surgery department. Mardini was excited for what lay ahead and thrilled that Nauta would push so hard for him.

It was a busy all-nighter in the cardiac intensive care unit. Talking with a colleague, Mardini learned that the newly formed integrated plastic surgery program of the medical school was looking to fill a space left by someone who had withdrawn. Although Mardini felt he had no interest in plastic surgery, he admired a professor teaching in the program, Christopher Attinger. "He did a lot of really cool things—including major reconstructions of various parts of the body—and he was so passionate about what he did," he said.

Half jokingly, Mardini wondered aloud to his friend, "What about me?" Ten minutes later, Attinger called Mardini to ask about his interest in the position. Having gotten no sleep the night before and now looking at the possibility of transitioning to a field he had never really considered before, Mardini found the whole experience a bit surreal. Attinger described the intense, lifesaving work plastic surgeons could do. Plastic surgery wasn't only about injecting Botox, doing liposuction, and performing breast augmentation, he said. In the two subspecialties that most interested Mardini, craniofacial surgery and reconstructive microsurgery, surgeons shaped heads, restored facial features, reconstructed body parts, and changed lives.

Attinger arranged for Mardini to speak with Scott Spear, founding chair of the Department of Plastic Surgery at Georgetown. Spear, a plastic surgeon who pioneered breast reconstruction and had published hundreds of articles and books, soon offered Mardini the vacancy in the plastic surgery program. Mardini felt torn. The opportunity was undeniably fascinating, and the position a hard one to get, but accepting it would change his vision of his career. Plastic surgery was appealing because it offered the opportunity to do work that was complex, life-enhancing, and lifesaving. He could interact with individual patients over many years and treat a variety of conditions, including cleft lip and palate, facial injuries, congenital disorders, and wounds all over the body.

Yet Mardini still loved pediatric cardiac surgery. He delayed for weeks while deciding whether to accept the offer. At last Mardini figured he could always go back to cardiac surgery if he really wanted to, so he dove into plastic surgery. He transitioned from cracking chests and massaging hearts to operating on small hand lesions and more complex upper extremity reconstructions. He was now operating at the Curtis National Hand Center at Union Memorial Hospital in Baltimore, where Georgetown University plastic surgery residents received their experience in hand surgery, a branch of plastic surgery.

The shift from the intensity of cardiac surgery to the minute scale of hand surgery felt jarring at times. Mardini sometimes wondered if he had made a mistake by changing direction. If he was going to be a plastic surgeon, he wanted the work to be intense, and so far he had not experienced the thrill he had glimpsed during his general surgery residency and cardiac surgery rotations. Sometimes he felt lost in his new specialty. Even his father was not enthusiastic about the change. To counteract his stress and frustration, Mardini poured his free hours into exercising and running.

During his final year in the plastic surgery program, Mardini began investigating fellowships in two different fields: craniofacial surgery, which focused on craniofacial bony structures and lip and palate, and reconstructive microsurgery, which involved reconstructing all parts of the body, including transplanting tissues from one part of the body to another. These, he determined, were the subspecialties within plastic surgery that could deliver the high-adrenaline, high-stakes rush he sought.

Mardini soon learned of an intriguing microsurgery fellowship in Taiwan with a renowned surgeon named Fu-Chan Wei, who excelled in surgery, teaching, speaking, and leading his program. He was a legendary figure at the Chang Gung Memorial Hospital Microsurgery Center in Taoyuan City, about twenty miles from Taipei, the capital of Taiwan.

Few Americans went to Taiwan for medical study, but this did not deter Mardini from considering it. Two of his surgical mentors, giants in the fields of reconstructive surgery and craniofacial surgery, Attinger and Jeffrey Posnick, urged him to give serious thought to studying at Chang Gung. After talking over his options with a friend, Mardini decided he would go to Taiwan if he could somehow arrange to become a double fellow in both reconstructive microsurgery and craniofacial surgery at Chang Gung. It seemed an unlikely prospect, as Wei did not favor the idea of having a fellow in two specialties. But Mardini and his medical advisors eventually prevailed, and Chang Gung offered him six months of training in each specialty.

Many of Mardini's professional acquaintances had hoped he would accept a fellowship in the United States. His parents wondered why he wanted to stray so far from his close-knit family. When they gathered in Washington to see him off at the airport, his mother shed some tears, a sight Mardini had not witnessed before. Still, Mardini held to his decision and focused on keeping his spirits positive.

Mardini arrived in Taiwan on a Friday in July 2001, with his flight landing at 5:00 a.m. After heading to the hospital and finding his living quarters, he put on scrubs and met with the surgeons he would be working with. One of the first people he met was Hung-Chi Chen, an accomplished reconstructive microsurgeon who would later become one of Mardini's main mentors and dear friends. Hung-Chi offered Mardini the chance to start with reconstructive microsurgery but was also open to Mardini's preference for starting with the craniofacial fellowship.

Mardini then met plastic surgeon Philip Chen, and they discussed the details of the fellowship. He advised Mardini to go home, relax, and return on Monday morning. However, Mardini declined, eager to stay and experience a typical surgical day. They ended up operating late into the evening. Around 11:00 p.m., as they were wrapping up a surgery, Mardini asked a nurse where Philip was so he could say goodbye. To his surprise, Philip was starting another surgery in a different room, which continued until 1:30 a.m.

As they were finishing up, Mardini inquired about Philip's weekend plans. Philip mentioned he would be in the clinic on Saturday starting at 8:00 a.m., following a 7:00 a.m. conference, but assured Mardini he didn't need to attend. Nonetheless, Mardini decided to go to the 7:00 a.m. conference and then join Philip at the clinic. To his astonishment, they spent the entire day, from 8:00 a.m. to 8:00 p.m., seeing 120 patients. Although the discussions were in Mandarin and Taiwanese—languages unfamiliar to Mardini—Philip graciously explained each patient's problems, treatment plans, and possibilities.

That day, Mardini realized he had come to a remarkable place for training. The surgeons were legendary for a reason—they were not only exceptional educators but also outstanding surgeons. Mardini recognized how fortunate he was to have this opportunity and was determined to make the most of it.

The environment at Chang Gung was incredibly busy and intense, but the hospital was also a bastion of educational excellence. Mardini's mind was whirling excitedly. Chang Gung had four thousand beds and was one of five hospitals on an enormous medical campus. Thirty of its ICU beds and seventy of its hospital beds were dedicated to plastic surgery. The plastic surgery team worked on cancers of the head and neck, reconstructions, trauma, cleft lip and palate, cranial vault reshaping, jaw surgery, and much else. Mardini had never seen anything like it.

He soon fell in with the people he was going to be working with in microsurgery and craniofacial surgery, people who operated every day, all day. He began in craniofacial surgery working with Philip Chen, who frequently did ten to fifteen surgeries in a day, one after another. In the mornings Mardini often attended the craniofacial clinic, where more than a hundred patients awaited treatment every day. He then operated until late at night. It promised to be a complete immersion in the specialty, absorbing and relentless, a happy dream come true for Mardini.

After a week of exhilarating work, Mardini at last had a chance to meet Fu-Chan Wei for the first time. The head plastic surgeon delivered upsetting news: he insisted that Mardini could complete only one fellowship there after all. Doing both would be impossible—a separation of focus that Wei wanted his fellows to avoid. Mardini protested that he had passed over other opportunities to come to Taiwan with the assurance that doing two fellowships there would be possible. Wei remained unmoved. The following week, he said, Mardini would have to choose between craniofacial surgery and microsurgery.

When they met again, Wei had researched Mardini's situation. He acknowledged that Mardini's two fellowships had been approved, although in error, while Wei was away from the hospital. Nonetheless, he agreed to give Mardini a one-time, exclusive exemption to the one-fellowship rule. Mardini's stay in Taiwan was extended to eighteen months and later extended again, so that he could complete the training in both specialties. Wei and Mardini would eventually publish a textbook on reconstructive surgery together.

What followed was a demanding fellowship schedule in which Mardini thrived. He moved between performing a range of procedures—from esophageal reconstructions to transplants of toes as finger replacements—and consultations, surgeries at remote hospitals, and meetings with colleagues. There was little time for leisure or even sleep. He would start his day at 7:00 a.m. and end it between 3:00 and 4:00 a.m., a schedule he could maintain because he had only himself to worry about. Every day the same taxi driver would pick him up and bring him home to his small apartment.

Five years passed, and Mardini gave little consideration to returning to the United States. He was where he wanted to be, and he was willing to pursue his passions and interests wherever they might take him. He was learning so much and gaining so much valuable experience that he did not want to leave yet. He met visiting microsurgeons and craniofacial surgeons from around the world. He had also learned to speak some Mandarin. "What I had there was amazing to me," he said. True, he was removed from family and friends, but "being in Taiwan was just the best thing ever." When he speculated about leaving, he thought he would go to the East or West Coast of the United States. The vast and vague territory in between was beyond his reckoning.

Those thoughts remained speculations until 2005, when a friend he had met during his plastic surgery residency, Steven Moran, now working at Mayo Clinic, mentioned they had a position open in Rochester, Minnesota. Mardini thought there was no way he would relocate to the Midwest. He did not know much about the area, and he did not want to know. Moran countered that during a forthcoming trip back to the United States to visit his parents on the East Coast, Mardini could stop at Mayo Clinic on the way.

So Mardini came to Rochester, visited Mayo, and found himself in a job interview. "I was almost not believing that was really happening," he said. The idea of continuing his career in such an out-of-the-way place as Minnesota seemed ridiculous, but he felt mesmerized by what he was learning about Mayo. He met several of the Mayo plastic surgeons. The campus seemed clean and modern, although many of its buildings were decades old.

When Mardini returned to Taiwan, he dove back into his work but soon heard again from Mayo. Would he come back for a second interview? His Minnesota hosts said he had not met everyone the first time.

He returned in January 2006. Arriving on a Sunday in the dead of winter, Mardini checked into a hotel in Rochester, and at 9:00 p.m. found himself, groggy and jet-lagged, ironing a shirt for his meeting the next morning with a contingent of Mayo physicians. "There was nobody around," he remembered. "It felt sad and lonely." He seemed to be in the middle of nowhere, in a cold place where the sun set too early in the day. But his prospective colleagues did their best to dispel this perspective. They engaged and intrigued him during meetings and interviews the next day.

Spending time with the plastic surgery group, Mardini began to appreciate the distinctiveness of Mayo Clinic, its special relationship with patients, its spirit of collaboration among doctors and staff, and its philosophy of always putting patients' needs first. He started to grasp a unique feature of the Mayo environment— that the institution valued collegiality, friendliness, and openness to constructive criticism. He met a variety of people he might team up with at Mayo: thoracic surgeons, general surgeons, oral and maxillofacial surgeons, orthopedic surgeons, and neurosurgeons. Finally, the group of plastic surgeons and their spouses, including former department chair and renowned surgeon P. G. Arnold, hosted Mardini for dinner at the Foundation House, the former home of one of the founding Mayo brothers. It was an overwhelming courtship. He felt honored by the warmth and welcome they gave him. Mardini left feeling it was possible he could live and succeed there.

A few days later, the Mayo hiring group offered Mardini the job. If he accepted it, his Mayo friend breezily suggested, Mardini could set up Mayo's face transplant program. That comment wedged itself in Mardini's mind, although at that point only one face transplant had been performed anywhere in the world. Mardini deliberated for two weeks. At a place like Mayo Clinic, he could work on his own big cases with the support of a strong institution and fantastic colleagues. He could advance his career, easily take time to visit his family, and travel for fun. The privilege of the offer sank in. "So I moved to Rochester," he said. He accepted a furnished apartment in a building that he lived in for the next fourteen years. Most weekends, he flew east to visit his family. He was single and free to do what he wanted.

After his initial orientation at Mayo, Mardini waded in. As part of a department of eight plastic surgeons, he was expected to work a full schedule seeing patients, attending meetings, and taking on various responsibilities. Shirley Walter, a senior office manager in the department, was asked to get Mardini up to speed until she felt he was able to work with a medical secretary and administrative support person with less experience than Walter had.

Mardini was always up and about, and Walter often had trouble finding him during his unexpectedly frequent visits with his patients. Mardini and Walter hit it off well, and she took a motherly approach to helping him get settled in his new position. Socializing was not high on Mardini's priority list, and he was generally a private man. But Walter wondered at times if he might be lonely. Mardini's Mayo colleagues immediately saw in him someone who was friendly, highly talented in his medical specialty, and easy to work with. His willingness to accept suggestions was striking and well matched to Mayo's embrace of teamwork. He projected confidence and seemed never to get upset with others.

Right away, Mardini started performing reconstructions and aesthetic surgery—whatever came his way. Two months into his new job, he was scheduled to be on call on Christmas Day, 2006, since new staff always received the least desirable assignments. That was when he met Andy Sandness.

When Andy arrived at Saint Marys, he was unconscious, in an induced coma. His face was disastrously wounded, blasted open.

Mardini had been brought in for consultation, and he could see the work that was ahead. "First you start to debride, or remove dead tissue, and clean out the wounds to prevent massive infections," Mardini said of the initial treatments. "You do two or three or four surgeries, just cleaning up the debris in his face. Next you start to bring the bones together with small plates and screws. The defect becomes smaller and the face takes on more of a normal structure. But with so much tissue missing, full normalcy is far from a reality." In the days that followed, more tissue died. "You wait two or three days, and you go back in again. We did that—I haven't counted, but I'm guessing eight to fifteen times over a two-week period."

Mardini's private appraisal of the new patient was that there was practically no structure left to Andy's face. Andy was noseless and drooling, with his unrestrained tongue hanging out. Mardini had performed surgeries on people with cancers that left major deformities, but mid-face injuries, as Andy had experienced, were unusual. "I was trying to figure out whether to do even anything for this patient," Mardini remembers. "I didn't remember a similar [patient] in the past. What am I supposed to do?" Dozens of surgeries loomed ahead. Could the patient accept and endure the treatment? Intricate structures such as the eyelids, nose, tongue, teeth, and mouth, along with their supporting drainage systems, were notoriously difficult to reconstruct.

Once Andy was out of immediate danger, Mardini began to consider how to create the basic foundation of a reconstructed face that could offer a functional, if not fully normal, life. Given the sobering degree of Andy's injury, Mardini was not certain he could achieve that goal for Andy. In addition, Mardini found it challenging to communicate with his new patient. "It's very hard to get to know someone who's missing a face," he said, noting Andy's inability to speak.

Mardini was realistic about Andy's facial reconstruction. He believed it would take ten to fifteen surgeries to bring Andy to a reconstructed result in which he was not drooling and his face could perform basic functions. After another ten to fifteen surgeries, he might look like a patient who has been successfully reconstructed. Mardini foresaw "a lot of surgery, a lot of fear, [and] a lot of work, with a final outcome that's going to be disappointing," he said. He believed Andy would emerge better than he had been before the reconstruction process began, but his face would still appear disfigured. In other words, reconstruction came with significant shortcomings.

In one conversation, one in which Andy had a premonition that Mardini would bring bad news, the plastic surgeon told Andy that a new nose could be reconstructed but would require six to eight surgeries. Tissue from his forearm would be transplanted as a flap to provide the inner lining of the nose, transferred cartilage would create structure and stability, and tissue from the forehead would provide the exposed outer lining. The forehead flap would need two or three surgical thinnings, maybe more, to achieve the final outcome. The other option available to Andy would be to wear a prosthetic nose that could be glued or clipped onto his face.

The number of stages and surgeries required to reconstruct Andy's nose seemed overwhelming. Andy's mother, who was present at this consultation, began squeezing her son's hand tightly, too tightly, as she took in the doctor's words. It was dispiriting news. "She [was] just crushing my hand," Andy remembered. "She [was] devastated, and I thought, 'Mom, you're squeezing my hand so hard.'"

After this conversation, Rhonda followed Mardini out into the hallway. She needed assurance Andy would be treated as well as possible. She made Mardini pinky-promise, locking their little fingers, to take care of Andy. "To my mom, that was the world. That [promise] meant everything," Andy said. "She came back in, and she was relieved."

Rhonda tried to make the most of the limited time she could stay with Andy at Mayo. Often accompanied by her Wyoming friend Kim Fulton, Rhonda would carry around a small tape recorder in consultations with Andy's doctors. She used it to dictate her thoughts and remember the most important information that Andy's physicians told her.

"She is clearly distraught and overridden with emotion," one of the doctors wrote in Andy's medical record. Concerned about her well-being, the physician noted that she might benefit from emotional guidance. In fact, Rhonda had been walking around the hospital searching for a chapel. She had stopped attending her Baptist church in Newcastle months earlier, but now she wanted a place to pray.

The physician also worried that Rhonda's limited financial means made it impossible for her to remain long in Rochester, compounding her stress. The hotel room that Mayo's staff had reserved for her proved too expensive, and a social worker worried that "the family was currently driving around downtown with nowhere to go, and no resources." The family's chihuahua, which Rhonda had brought with her to Rochester, complicated the search for housing. Rhonda was keeping Andy's brother, Ronald, informed of Andy's condition, but she had not stayed in touch with Andy's father, Reed.

Mardini was leading Andy through an explanation of the forthcoming reconstruction process, slowly, step by step. All reconstructive plastic surgeons have their own approaches, and Mardini's was to maintain a positive outlook. Instead of telling Andy he would never return to his previous appearance, he emphasized that Andy could do well, make strides, and see improvement. He assured Andy that the next surgery would accomplish something important, and the one after that would concentrate on other improvements. He told Andy the process would be exhausting but that he would recover. And he broke recovery into small milestones.

Mardini made sure to communicate all steps with Andy and his family. Despite Mardini's concentration on the surgical aspects of Andy's facial reconstruction, he was aware of the social consequences of Andy's injury. It had left Andy and his mother psychologically traumatized, and there was the worrisome possibility that another suicide attempt might follow. Mardini realized that the despair and depression that Andy had felt before his suicide attempt could be worse after he saw his devastating injuries and understood their full import. Would Andy go through a long series of reconstructive surgeries only to attempt suicide again? As a new member of Mayo's medical staff who was about to commit himself and the institution to the major reconstruction that Andy needed, Mardini felt a responsibility to Mayo Clinic as well as to Andy. He did not want to travel too far down a particular road with a patient who might not bear up well under all the pressure of what was still to come.

To maximize Andy's recovery and to better inform his own decisions, Mardini brought Mayo's psychiatric staff onto Andy's team early on. Psychiatrist Scott Albin first met with Andy a few days after Andy arrived at the hospital. Albin noted seeing Andy intubated, with a cloth covering his face. Sedated and groggy, Andy could not communicate. At one point, the cloth was removed to change his dressings. The psychiatrist took note of the extreme injuries to Andy's face. "Part of his jaw is gone. I can make out seeing part of his cranial base in the inner parts of his nasal cavity and sinuses as if he has been filleted open," Albin wrote in the patient's medical record. The sight was sobering even for a seasoned physician. Once Andy's mind cleared, "one could only speculate about the possibility that he would not want to have medical surgical treatment," Albin wrote. He worried that Andy, in despair, might decline reconstructive surgery.

Albin also interviewed Andy's mother for her perspective on Andy's history. Soon after came psychiatric interviews with Andy. Albin's assessment of Andy, along with medical research on people who attempt suicide and severely injure themselves, convinced Albin that a good outcome was possible for Andy. It also helped assure Mardini that despite Andy's severe injuries, a repeat of the suicide attempt was unlikely, and Mardini could proceed with the extensive reconstruction of Andy's face.

At this point in Andy's treatment, he was often awake and alert, able to communicate by writing. He said his pain was well controlled. He could breathe well without a ventilator. His facial wounds no longer bled and were not infected. Although Andy was still receiving nutrients through his gastrostomy tube, he was now also swallowing small amounts of liquids. "I see no issues at this time that would require ongoing ICU care," a physician wrote in Andy's record.

Andy was receiving a variety of medications. They included an antibiotic ointment for his injured eyes, an antidepressant, pain medications, antibiotic salve for his forehead lacerations, a laxative, medication for agitation and nausea, antiseptic swabs for his damaged tongue, and a sleeping aid.

~

Andy had now spent a great deal of time in Mardini's company. He was beginning to learn about his doctor's personality and approach to medicine. "He's just selfless," Andy said in one of many interviews he later gave for this book. "He really is about helping people. It's not a job for him—he loves it. He seriously loves to help people."

Rhonda, who so far had been serving as Andy's decision-maker and communicator with the medical staff, planned to return to Newcastle on January 5, and Andy's sister, Rhiannon, had to leave soon after. Mayo's social workers kept in touch with Rhonda after her departure. On the phone, she was often tearful and described her struggles to pay bills and her frustration at being away from Andy's side. She also discussed with them Andy's lack of medical insurance and the costs that Mayo had so far been bearing. Although he had been working full-time at Statewide Electric at the time he shot himself, he had not made it through the six-month waiting period to become eligible for employer-provided medical insurance.

One of Mardini's strengths is gathering skilled people around him to care for his patients. He could accomplish that best if Andy moved out of the surgical intensive care unit at Saint Marys and to Mardini's own plastic surgery unit at the nearby Mayo Clinic Hospital, Methodist Campus, the other of Mayo's two hospitals in Rochester. The transfer happened on January 5, the same day Andy's mother was to leave for Wyoming. Andy's sister and mother met him in his new room. Through writing, he assured them he was not in significant pain.

Andy began receiving psychiatric care from Gayla Tennen around this time. One of the first questions the psychiatrist had pondered was when Andy should look at his face. Rhonda had hoped to be with Andy when he got his first look. Tennen wanted Andy to take the initiative. "He has not expressed a desire to view his injuries as of yet," she wrote. "I think it would be detrimental to do so before he expresses readiness." She recommended a sensitive and cautious approach to this momentous unveiling, which could set the tone for Andy's recovery. If it was done too early, she feared, Andy might feel repelled and ashamed of his image for a long time to come.

At a meeting with Tennen in early January, Andy was awake, alert, and watching television. He had come to a decision. He told Tennen, writing on his whiteboard, that he had looked at his bandaged face in a mirror and knew his face was "really deformed right now," he wrote. "I don't like it, but at least I am alive." He also affirmed his willingness to begin the long process of facial reconstructive surgery.

On January 12, 2007, in a follow-up meeting with Tennen, Andy assured her that his earlier suicidal thoughts had not returned. He characterized his current mood as "OK." Tennen discussed with him the possibility of discontinuing the one-to-one care he was receiving. One-to-one care ensured that a caregiver was always nearby to watch over him. Under standard nursing care, there would be times when his caregivers were not in his room and would be caring for other patients. Andy would live in a private room, as he had since his initial admission.

Andy said he would be happy with standard nursing care. Tennen explained the importance of keeping him safe, including safe from himself, but his denial of suicidal intent persuaded her. She recommended an end to his one-on-one care but cautioned in her notes that "the estimation of risk is an imperfect process. If he were to exhibit a change of behavior [or] anxiety, agitation or distress, or voice any suicidal thoughts, one-to-one care should be restarted without delay." One-to-one care was never needed or restarted, but the next few weeks of reconstructive surgery would test Andy's resilience.

# Chapter 4

# Looking in the Mirror

———

The human face serves a multitude of physiological purposes, but its psychological and social roles are just as important. Members of only a few animal species besides humans can recognize their own faces—gorillas, elephants, magpies, and bottlenose dolphins. Humans scrutinize their faces, decorate them, pierce them, sometimes regard them critically, and above all depend on them to identify one another. Because the face is so important, facial disfigurement can deeply alter a person's life.

Physicians throughout history have worked to treat their patients' head and face injuries. Nearly three thousand years ago, Sushruta, a scholar and surgeon from Varanasi, India, described how to attach a slice of skin from a patient's cheek to the nose, accomplishing an early form of rhinoplasty. In a manuscript, Sushruta also explained the use of a pedicle—a temporary lifeline of skin that kept the patch nourished with blood from the cheek—to keep the graft from dying, and he told how a damaged ear could be repaired using the same technique.

In 1597, when a teacher in Bologna, Italy, Gaspare Tagliacozzi, wrote of the use of a similar method to provide physical and psychological comfort to facially disfigured patients, the Catholic Church excommunicated him. If God saw fit to create or change the appearance of a person in a particular way, the Church maintained, it was sinful for humans to interfere. For centuries, reconstructive skin grafts fell from favor in Europe and were ridiculed as fantasy.

A small number of surgeons persisted, but they ran into a serious limitation: any living tissue used to repair a facial injury had to originate with the patient. Using tissue from another person or an animal did not work, and only in the twentieth century did scientists discover why. The recipient's immune system would attack the grafted tissue with antibodies, causing pain, inflammation, and ultimately necrosis, or cellular death, in the affected tissue. This response, while essential in keeping the body protected from external viruses, bacteria, and other infectious agents, also makes grafts from beyond a patient's own body highly dangerous. Nothing, it seemed, could overcome the body's refusal to accept tissue from another source.

This barrier persisted well into the twentieth century. Many of the tragic battlefield disfigurements of World War I thus required the talents of artists, not surgeons, who crafted lifelike masks and other prosthetics for the facially wounded when the skills of physicians reached their limit. One such artist, the American sculptor Anna Coleman Ladd, was inspired by the work of the English artist Francis Derwent Wood to create beautifully painted copper and foil masks to cover the shot-off jaws, charred noses, and scarred eye sockets of the nearly one hundred French soldiers who visited her Red Cross Studio for Portrait Masks in Paris. "If the wounded man was blind, the mask would be equipped with artificial eyes,"

Ladd said years later. "Eyelashes, eyebrows, and even mustaches were affixed in the masks. They were light and durable. The masks will last a lifetime." The impact of Ladd's work was such that in 1932 the government of France made Ladd a Chevalier of the Legion of Honor.

At the time, it seemed that medicine could not help many of the most grievously injured. Still, several wartime doctors managed to advance reconstructive surgery despite the roadblocks thrown up by the human body's defenses. Among the many military hospitals the British established to treat injured soldiers, Queen's Hospital in Kent distinguished itself with a specialty in the new discipline of plastic surgery, which treated facial and jaw injuries. As the *Westminster Gazette* newspaper explained to readers new to that medical specialty, "The science of plastic surgery implies the building up of the features and restoration of contour from the patient's own tissues. Portions of skin, bone, and cartilage are today transferred and manipulated in a manner which a few months ago was regarded as an impossibility."

The surgeon Major Harold Gillies, a native of New Zealand, is the most famous of several doctors who launched remarkable advancements in plastic surgery at Queen's Hospital. An initial group of 310 soldiers, all bearing grievous facial wounds, were early beneficiaries. Before their treatments, fellow soldiers uncomfortably avoided them. Members of the group felt isolated. For these patients, Gillies used grafts from the inside of their mouths to build new lips and grafted face patches from other parts of their bodies. The results were functional but not always aesthetically pleasing.

Another of Gillies's patients, a sailor named Walter Yeo, who had been disfigured in 1916 during the Battle of Jutland, received a grafted skin patch to cover a large wound in the center of his face. To nourish the newly grafted skin, which had originated on Yeo's chest, Gillies extended pedicles like those Sushruta had described millennia earlier. The reporter who observed Gillies wrote, "A revolution has come. A new face is grafted on, and grows there, and becomes a real face—not a mask that hides horror." The procedure was plagued by infections that were hard to dampen, but Yeo eventually recovered so fully that he was able to return to naval service three years after his injury. He lived to the age of seventy.

Amazingly, the miracle of facial reconstruction had grown from the ugliness of war. After World War I was over, Gillies continued to perfect his techniques. In 1930, newspapers reported on the case of a schoolboy from Skegness, Luke Foster, whose nose had been malformed since birth. Using skin grafted from the boy's body, Gillies crafted a new nose that dramatically improved Foster's appearance and even allowed him to blow his nose for the first time. Later that year, King George V knighted Gillies for his medical efforts.

During World War II, another New Zealander and a cousin of Gillies's, the plastic surgeon Archibald McIndoe, treated hundreds of burned and facially wounded service members at Queen Victoria Hospital in East Grinstead, West Sussex, England. One of McIndoe's patients, an airman named Paul Hart, was blinded and badly burned on his face in a plane crash. He told doctors he wished he would die. McIndoe promised Hart he would help him recover, and over many months of reconstructive surgeries the pilot regained ears, a nose, lips, and his eyesight.

Another of McIndoe's patients, Ross Stewart, could not bear to look at himself in a mirror when he was admitted to the hospital. He needed a reconstructed nose, chin, lips, and eyelids, and it took thirty-six operations to reconstruct his face. But Stewart successfully endured the treatments and later enrolled in medical school. Through such experiences, McIndoe felt that his job was not only to repair faces and bodies but also to treat the spirits of those who believed their situations were hopeless. McIndoe, too, earned a knighthood for his work.

In 1931, a group of surgeons in the United States created the American Society of Plastic and Reconstructive Surgery. Soon after, in 1937, Mayo Clinic established its own plastic surgery residency program. By the 1950s, most facial reconstruction surgeries were performed on civilians, not members of the military. When Andy Sandness arrived at Mayo Clinic in 2006, Mayo had been training plastic surgeons for nearly seventy years.

January 15 marked Andy's first extensive reconstructive operation. Mardini and his plastic surgery team began by reconstructing Andy's lower jawbone using bone and tissue harvested from the fibula of his left leg. Recovery was painful and difficult. A temporary boost in pain medication left Andy too groggy to use his whiteboard to communicate. Feeling distressed, he lashed out when receiving treatment or having to move. Because of the harvested bone, he limped on his left leg and complained of numbness in his toes. Over the next week, Andy resisted walking, and sometimes refused to try. "Does not make eye contact when spoken to," a staff member recorded. Withdrawn, he refused to allow nurses to open his swollen left eye to check his vision and was unable to open it without their aid.

Psychiatrist Gayla Tennen caught up with Andy in his room on January 23. She asked how he was feeling. "Fine," Andy wrote on the whiteboard. He felt pain, but it was diminishing. Then he volunteered that he was tired of "sitting around." He now wanted to move more and wrote that he was willing to receive more physical therapy to get himself moving. He said he didn't feel depressed, anxious, or a sense of worthlessness or hopelessness, but he felt guilty about putting his family through the suicide ordeal and became visibly upset as he mentioned his feelings of guilt. He insisted that he would not try to harm himself again in the future.

Two weeks after his first reconstruction surgery, Andy underwent another. This time Mardini concentrated on Andy's damaged left orbital bone and cheekbone. He repaired several bone fractures using tiny plates and screws. During recovery, Andy received therapy to improve the range of motion in his reconstructed jaw. Andy's brother, Ronald, stayed with him during part of his recovery.

Over the next few weeks, Andy made substantial progress. He said he felt more like himself than at any time since his hospital admission. He was sleeping and able to concentrate and read normally, and he was comfortable walking long distances.

When Tennen brought up the sensitive subject of looking at his own unbandaged face in a mirror, Andy replied that he had avoided it and did not expect to see himself fully until after another round of reconstructive facial surgery. He had gazed at his own eyes in a mirror, had caught a glimpse of his chin, but had not seen the central part of his face at all. When he thought ahead to leaving the hospital and returning to Newcastle, presumably to live with his mother, he expected to be a recluse. He didn't think he would want to show his face around town. "He has been afraid to look because he is not sure how he would react to seeing himself in this condition," observed another psychiatrist, who called Andy's reluctance "a major concern" and "what could almost be considered a phobic response to looking at the major destruction of his face."

In the next reconstructive operation, on February 6, Mardini cut dead tissue from Andy's facial wounds, repaired fractures of his right cheekbone, and used skin from Andy's leg to reconstruct a lower lip. Grafted skin usually grows blood vessels and connects to the surrounding tissue within a few days. A wound remains at the donor site from which the skin originally came, and healing occurs more slowly than at the new location of the grafted skin. The wound at the donor site is often painful, requiring pain medication, and it can take weeks to heal. A week after the February 6 operation, Andy returned to surgery for a reconstruction of his upper jaw using a bone graft from the iliac crest, the upper part of his pelvis.

With his lower jaw and palate not yet fully reconstructed, Andy still could not readily communicate using his voice. Although he could vocalize with his tracheostomy plugged or unplugged, his speech was difficult to understand because of his severe facial injuries, and it was still painful for Andy to speak, so he continued to rely on the whiteboard to communicate. A speech pathologist recommended speech therapy once Andy's reconstruction progressed further.

A CT scan of Andy's head and face on March 13 detailed Andy's gains from reconstruction. The large soft tissue opening in the center of his face was now partly closed. The fibular grafts were starting to fuse with his lower jaw. Titanium mesh reinforced his left orbital floor. Implanted fasteners bolstered his reconstructed upper jaw. Still remaining in his face were bullet fragments and injuries to the floor of his mouth.

The two earlier grafts of tissue and bones from one part of the body to another held fast. They helped Andy achieve the functional outcomes his team wanted: a lessening of drooling and the ability to keep food in his mouth and swallow it. His most recent reconstructive surgeries improved his ability to speak. Surgically created flaps also measured as successes. They healed to surrounding tissues and made Andy's face more functional.

During successive surgeries, Mardini adhered skin to Andy's upper jaw, closed his upper lip, and reconstructed his chin. The rifle shot had blasted open Andy's eyelid, and Mardini used a combination of sutures and wires to gather its edges back to where they belonged. Additional accomplishments included repair of Andy's lower lip and grafting new tissue for the sides of his mouth and a nasal airway.

Andy's teeth also needed attention. Thomas Salinas, a prosthodontist at Mayo, examined Andy early on, and medical records indicate that Salinas was taken aback by Andy's appearance. At the time, Andy had not yet undergone any reconstruction to his face, and because of his tracheostomy, "he couldn't really talk, and actually didn't want to," Salinas remembers. "He would nod in understanding [at] what I was saying, but that was really about it."

Andy's 3D CT scan and a panoramic X-ray showed significant structural damage to his mouth. A fragment of his upper jaw still held three teeth. Two molars clung to the reconstructed part of his lower jaw. Salinas, who had come from Louisiana State University some years before to contribute to Mayo's century-long tradition of dentistry working in cooperation with medicine, recommended a bone graft to replace the fragment of the lower jaw that held the molars. He also began thinking about a prosthesis for Andy to replace his absent nose. Before making a recommendation for a prosthetic nose, however, Salinas wanted to see Andy's progress with facial reconstruction.

Once Mardini performed the bone graft and reconstruction of Andy's upper jaw and upper lip, Salinas felt confident about proceeding with the design of a prosthetic nose. It would help solve the flow of mucus coming down his nasal cavities, as well as improve his appearance. Salinas made an impression of the center of Andy's face using a hydrocolloid elastic, a kind of material that morphs from liquid to semisolid with the flexibility to be set and removed from the oral and nasal areas without damaging the tissues. The material was applied to the face from Andy's lower eye orbits to his chin. Salinas used the mold to create a wax model and finally sculpt a silicone prosthesis with a solid fit to Andy's face. The goal was to give Andy a transitional artificial nose—one that would work for him until future prostheses could be created and made usable. A well-designed prosthetic nose would allow Andy the prospect of eventually getting back to work and returning to his community.

~

In a little over two months, Andy had undergone reconstructive facial surgery multiple times. It was an exhausting ordeal that sometimes left him with little energy for anything other than healing. The hospital provided Andy with a TTY telephone, which used texting technology to allow people with speech disabilities to communicate with others. He also had a computer to send and receive emails. When a social worker asked Andy if he was using those devices to keep in touch with friends and family, he said he was. Nurses confirmed, though, that he had used the TTY phone only to communicate with his mother in Newcastle, and he hadn't used the computer at all.

Next, a social worker brought up with him the possibility of going home to Newcastle for a couple of weeks before returning to Mayo for more reconstructive surgery. She outlined how Andy could take care of his own dressing changes and tube feedings while away. Andy's drug regimen, which included intravenous antibiotics, would require him to buy the medication and pay for limited home healthcare. Without medical insurance, Andy would be out at least $200 per day during his time away from Mayo Clinic. In the end, Andy decided not to return home, even for a short stay, because of the expense and his difficulty walking after his surgeries.

Andy's spirits rose when friends from Wyoming made the trek to Rochester to visit him. "For them to make that trip, and especially in the wintertime, it was hard," he said. But Andy also spent a lot of time in the hospital alone. "My mom couldn't make it up there, my brother had to pay bills. I understood completely. It sucks, being up there by yourself." He passed the time sleeping and watching hours of football and basketball on ESPN. He watched as much as he could of basketball player Kobe Bryant, a longtime favorite whose branded shoes Andy owned. "Kobe was my hero. . . . He was at the prime of his career then," Andy said. He especially appreciated Bryant's approach to playing. "If you have the mentality of 'I can do anything,' you can really do anything. . . . Never stop chasing your dreams." Years later, when Bryant died in a helicopter crash in 2020, Andy wept.

Andy's time in the hospital brought challenges to his family as well. Rhonda made periodic visits to Andy, sometimes with Andy's brother, Ronald. But the family often had nowhere to stay and sometimes spent extended hours in the hospital's lounges. The fact that Ronald's boss could not guarantee Ronald's job during extended absences added another layer of stress. Ronald's car had a broken heater, requiring him to set a lit candle on the dashboard to keep the windshield from frosting over in winter driving. Eventually a small heater that plugged into the cigarette lighter made the candle unnecessary. Ronald, frequently accompanied by Rhonda, drove covered with blankets. Andy appreciated his brother's appearances, in part in anticipation of the strawberry shakes Ronald would sneak in from Starbucks.

At the start of his hospitalization, Andy had politely turned down the hospital chaplains who offered to talk with him and lend spiritual assistance. By March, though, he was more open to a chaplain stopping by, perhaps because, as one chaplain observed, "he's here alone and says he doesn't expect any visitors." The chaplain began coming by regularly, although she was not certain of his religious beliefs. Together, they watched baseball games on TV. Andy talked with her about what returning home would be like. He had doubts about attending church, although the chaplain encouraged him to try it. "I asked him to consider finding a person who could be a spiritual companion for him," she noted, "someone who accepts him as he is and will be an honest friend to him. We talked about the time it takes for spiritual healing."

With Andy's release from the hospital nearing, his care team wanted to know how well he could take in and swallow food. Earlier he had been able to use a straw to drink, but what about eating soft solid food? In early April, imaging tests showed what happened when he tried to eat applesauce and a banana. He had difficulty managing the food in his reconstructed mouth and forming it into a swallowable mass, but once he accomplished this he could swallow normally. Although his efforts to chew a soft cookie failed, his care team believed his eating technique would improve.

April also brought a reduction in Andy's facial swelling that allowed Salinas to finish his work on the prosthetic nose. Salinas and Mardini repositioned trumpets designed to prevent obstruction in Andy's nasal passages. Salinas completed the wax model of Andy's new nose and selected a skin tone with Mardini's help. On April 18, Salinas did the final trimming and coloring of the prosthetic and presented it to Andy, who learned how to apply, remove, and clean it. When the chaplain congratulated Andy on his new nose, he replied that he suspected it looked nothing like his old nose, even though he had not yet actually looked at it on his face.

At last Andy seemed willing to confront his reluctance to look at his face. Although he was ready to leave the hospital to return to his family in Wyoming, he was anxious about appearing in public with his damaged face. His lifelong shyness and guardedness in expressing his emotions, he knew, would likely increase. He dreaded being stared at and judged for his face. "I knew they weren't going to let me out until I looked at my face, and I thought, 'I'm staying here forever, then,'" Andy recalled.

At the time, Andy began working with Mayo psychologist Autumn Braddock, who wanted him to consider a type of treatment called exposure therapy. This therapy was used to help people anticipating a return to society after suffering grievous visible injuries. She devised a plan that would edge him toward acceptance of his looks. "I explained how in reality his face is not dangerous, but that his anxiety surrounding it is preventing him from being able to look at it [and] moving forward," Braddock noted.

Andy admitted being fearful of his own and others' reactions to his face. He told of touching his bandages and feeling obvious changes in the shape of his chin, the absence of his nose, his missing teeth, and the altered bone structure around his eyes. Discussing his physical changes made him upset and regretful. He now realized he was loved and appreciated by his friends and family, and his suicide attempt had been a "major mistake," he said.

Braddock believed Andy would benefit from long-term mental health therapy in Wyoming that would allow him to forgive himself and reduce his anxiety. But he also needed help now, before he left the protective environment of Mayo Clinic. The exposure therapy she proposed for Andy advanced in six steps: talking about his face, imagining what it looked like, touching it, looking at pictures of part of his face, looking at actual portions of part of it, and, finally, looking at his entire reflection.

"I strongly urged him to consider looking at his face in this manner rather than engaging in a flooding experience where he looks at his entire face impulsively," Braddock noted. With diligence and fortitude from Andy, all of this could be accomplished before he left the hospital for Newcastle. Andy agreed to try it, on the condition that he would not look at his entire face until his nose prosthesis was ready to wear. He and Braddock decided to begin the exposure therapy the week of April 16.

In their first session together, Braddock took photos of Andy's face to use in future sessions. They discussed the rationale for exposure therapy, and Braddock instructed Andy on first exposing his eyes only. With the rest of his face covered, he was to look at his eyes in a mirror twice daily, preferably with other people present to encourage him in case he had difficulty completing the exposures. After each exposure and throughout the process, Braddock asked him to use a form to rate the anxiety he felt. She would meet with him again the next day to continue the therapy, and she planned to complete her work with Andy within a week.

In his hospital room, Andy did as Braddock suggested. With a towel covering all his face except his eyes, he looked at himself. His eyes stared back from the mirror. He initially felt anxious, but the feeling gradually faded.

Andy met with Braddock again the next day. Andy looked at the photos Braddock had taken of his partial profile. He absorbed them with difficulty. Nonetheless, he "was able to gain some acceptance as we progressed," Braddock observed. "He was able to note the good and bad in each of the pictures. He was able to acknowledge what parts of his face have remained intact and those that have been irreversibly damaged." Braddock asked Andy to continue the photo exposures on his own along with the exposures to his eyes. After each exposure, she advised him to distract himself by watching TV, playing on his computer, or talking with someone.

They met every day or two. As Andy moved up the six-step exposure ladder, he kept track of his anxiety levels, which gradually became milder. Andy stuck to Braddock's process even when he cleaned and readhered his prosthetic nose; he did so carefully, without looking in a mirror. Eventually he saw photos of his complete profile and front-view photos of his face.

On April 25, he was ready to look at his full face in the mirror. He was eager to do so, he said. Braddock advised him to stand eight feet back from the mirror. She removed a towel that was covering the mirror and let him view his face for two to three minutes. Her plan was to follow the exposure with a discussion of his emotional response. After describing what he was seeing, Andy sat down and began to cry.

"I will never be able to do the things that I wanted to do," Andy told her. "I am always going to be alone." He despaired for his future and happiness. He would always need to hide from people, he believed. Braddock had not seen him so distraught before. She assured Andy that his deeply felt response was to be expected, given that this was his first time seeing his disfigured face in full. She also pointed out that Andy was catastrophizing, thinking of his future in all-or-nothing terms. Although shooting himself was a decision he now regretted with all his heart, he had the opportunity to make new decisions that he could feel good about. He could resolve to keep up the exposure therapy and continue to live his life as he would like to, despite the way his face looked. Braddock gently reminded Andy that adjusting to his face and forgiving himself for his past mistakes was a process he had only just begun.

Andy's final session with Braddock was on April 26, just two days before his departure from the hospital. By then Andy had rallied. He'd gathered the inner strength he needed to complete five full facial exposures since the previous day. He moved closer to the mirror for each viewing. His anxiety dropped after successive exposures. He said his mirror image saddened him less and that his mood was better. He still worried about his future, but he felt a glimmer of acceptance and optimism about the life ahead of him. He was excited to be returning home and promised to work on overcoming his fear of others' reactions to his appearance. He planned to take a shower that day with the mirror uncovered, something he had avoided due to fear that he would catch a glimpse of himself. "I can't live in the shadows, and have to live my life," Andy said to Braddock. It was an emotional moment for both him and Braddock.

Although Andy had made progress, his concerns about his appearance persisted. He could now tolerate glances in the mirror, mainly to groom himself and apply and readjust his prosthetic nose, but he still avoided his reflection whenever possible. The exposure therapy technique helped, yet Andy found it difficult to truly accept his reconstructed appearance. "I didn't like who I was," he said. There seemed no way for him to completely overcome that feeling.

Andy told Braddock that once home in Newcastle, he planned to spend time with friends, get a dog, and find a part-time job. She cautioned him that he was bound to have some difficult days, and she gave him strategies to keep himself active and social. Braddock worried, however, that Andy had no mental health care set up in Newcastle. She referred him to providers there and set up an appointment to meet with Andy when he returned to Mayo in June for follow-up treatment. Braddock told Mardini about Andy's progress in viewing his face, which Mardini was pleased to hear.

Andy had spent more than four months at Mayo, and the reconstructive work was over, at least for the time being. Andy was weary of living in a hospital and wanted to move on. Yet he felt apprehensive about how people in Newcastle, his hometown, where everybody knew everything about everyone, would receive him with a reconstructed but still clearly damaged face.

Visible injury and malformation of the face produce deep psychological complications. And people who become disfigured as adults suffer the most. Andy's facial reconstruction helped his face appear no longer freshly wounded, but few would regard it without shock or at least curiosity. Andy anticipated some of the difficulties he would encounter back home, but he had no way of knowing how much his appearance would affect every aspect of his life outside the hospital, from making friends to communicating with others.

"Successful adaptation required individuals to change their personal value system and to place less reliance upon appearance," one psychological study of disfigurement concluded. Could Andy make that difficult adjustment?

In his final days before leaving Mayo, Andy thought constantly about how his life had changed course over the previous four months. "Every day, I realized my life was now so different," he said. "A lot of bad things happened, all that I did to my friends and family and myself." He found himself still feeling waves of guilt, regret, and anger at himself. Andy's care team asked for Rhonda's help in leading Andy to schedule a chemical dependence evaluation, refrain from using alcohol and other drugs, and find mental health therapy when he returned to Newcastle.

Andy was discharged from the hospital on April 30, 2007. He left with a small mouth, a nose that existed as a silicone attachment, only a few teeth remaining, dim vision in his left eye, and limited use of his tongue. On the other hand, 90 percent of his speech was now intelligible, and he could eat solid food with increasing confidence, although he still needed to break it up into small pieces before placing it in his mouth and slowly chewing it.

Ronald and one of Andy's friends had driven to Rochester from Newcastle, and they would take Andy home. Andy's Mayo nurses and other caregivers were sad to see him go after working with him for so long. He still wonders if they learned about what came later in his life. "I hope they did," he said.

Mardini believed that in many ways his patient had successfully come through the recent tumultuous months. Andy's facial reconstruction allowed him to eat on his own, swallow, and speak. The grafted tissues from his leg and hip to rebuild his upper and lower jaw had survived in their new locations on his face. The shattered bones had healed. Andy had benefited from the help of several psychiatrists involved in his case, and they would stay involved.

Andy showed great appreciation for what had been done for him. To others, "he never showed disappointment," Mardini said. "He never showed dissatisfaction."

But Andy's lack of expressed dissatisfaction, Mardini believed, did not amount to total success. Andy's face remained far from the average in function and appearance. Meeting him for the first time, you might wonder what you were looking at. Many people would be taken aback. After visiting Andy ten or twenty times, you could grow accustomed to his appearance, Mardini thought. But "I wasn't satisfied," he said. "I want to see a patient who's really happy and back to being normal." To edge closer to this goal, Mardini foresaw further reconstructive surgeries for Andy ahead.

# Chapter 5

# Homecoming

———

A ndy came home in late April, a time when the northeastern part of Wyoming typically sees temperatures in the fifties and sixties and sunny skies. He had spent the entire Northern Plains winter in a distant hospital almost entirely indoors. To an outdoorsman like Andy, confinement within walls was no gift, even in the Minnesota cold.

He spent his first night back in Rhonda's home. He felt bad about the effect of his suicide attempt on himself and his mother. He feared he had put her through a living hell and worried that the shock would forever affect her. "She was tough, so she never acted bothered," Andy said. But he knew his attempt to kill himself had devastated her. When she showed him the police report from the day of his injury, Andy apologized.

After that first night he often stayed with his brother, Ronald. Even so, mother and son remained close. They often spent time together, sometimes teaming up for outdoor barbeques.

Life in his hometown was different. Previously he would make carefree visits to the bar, take walks down the street, and go on casual shopping trips. Now he never went to restaurants—"never, ever," he said. He had to tear food into small pieces. Only with difficulty could he move food into his small mouth. Many foods—including breakfast cereal, soup, and pasta—fell out of his mouth as he tried to eat them. Because of his missing teeth and difficulty chewing, it was all too easy to choke on salads, nuts, and hard candies. Eating became a strictly private act for Andy. He did not like to be watched.

Many people with severe facial disfigurement feel the burden of social stigma as powerfully as they feel the disability of their functional limitations. "Most research shows that facial disfigurement results in lower self-confidence and a negative self-image that might persist throughout life," the authors of a 2018 study wrote in the *AMA Journal of Ethics*. Faces crucially figure into selection of a life partner, popularity, career choices, and character judgments. Because of this, some psychologists liken facial disfigurement to a kind of social death, resulting in a deep sense of grief for what was lost. People with such injuries frequently have a poor self-image, are confused about their identities, experience damage to relationships, and undergo bouts of mental illness.

Andy visited no other towns. He avoided making eye contact with others. When it was necessary for him to visit a store or other public place, he would not ask for help. If he needed something, he got it for himself. "I can handle it alone," was the message he told himself. "He became a recluse," Reed recalled.

His most inviolable personal law was that he would not gaze directly at children. The reconstructed features of his face—a mouth about an inch wide, no visible lips or teeth, facial bones at askew angles, a sunken chin, an artificial nose with discernible edges where it met his skin—often frightened them. Sometimes his nose fell off, and Andy would have to scramble on the ground to pick it up. He kept to himself, hidden in the house with Ronald, while Reed lived nearby in an attached apartment. He often visited Rhonda.

People in Newcastle knew he had tried to take his own life. Some wondered if he was safe to be around. "Everybody's judging," Andy said. "It's the way that we evolved, I guess. I don't know if we can see anybody for the way they are. We always want to be better than them."

On the occasions Andy ventured out, people often reacted to him by teasing, staring, commenting, and asking unsolicited questions. Everyone, it seemed, wanted to see what he looked like. "Some people will be jerks, others will be just inquisitive," Andy said. He noticed them looking. They gave him what he called "bad stares." "That hurt," Andy said. He did not believe any of them had a right to know the private details of his life, so he prepared various stories, such as telling people that he had been in a hunting accident. To get away, Andy took trips into the hills where he could be outdoors and fish with no prying eyes around.

Even his friends and neighbors, many of them prepared for a dramatic alteration of his appearance, had to reconcile the face they remembered as Andy's with the one he now had. The pre-gunshot Andy had had an oval face, a smooth and fleshy nose, and a wide mouth that often flashed into a large-toothed, broad smile. Not many people found the new Andy recognizable. Hell, Andy hardly recognized himself.

Not all his early experiences back home were negative. Many of his old friends tried to stick with and support him. He played baseball with buddies and loved it, even though he felt terribly out of shape. Unfortunately, swimming, which he used to enjoy, was now out of the question because he could not close his mouth and hold his breath. Going into deep water was potentially life-threatening.

~

People like Andy who receive reconstructive facial surgery can often gradually improve their self-esteem and partially resolve the acute discomfort they feel when they see themselves in a mirror. Andy, however, was not yet at that stage of recovery. He felt troubled that his surgeries had still left him with a visibly damaged face. He had to adapt to his prosthetic nose, the difficulties of eating with a small mouth, and his changed way of speaking. It was hard for him to express his emotions through facial expressions.

His prosthetic nose was a particularly challenging adjustment. One morning, Andy awoke in his mother's house to find his prosthetic nose missing. He typically removed it overnight and kept it on a nightstand, but it had vanished. Overcoming his reluctance to let Rhonda see him without the nose on, he told her what had happened. Andy, his mother, and Ronald searched the entire house. At last they found the prosthetic in the basement, where the family's chihuahua had hidden it. Andy believed the dog, who was fond of him, disliked seeing him wearing the nose. So the dog took it from Andy's bedroom, stashed it downstairs, and returned to cuddle with Andy in peace.

Over the next several years, Andy went through six or seven prosthetic noses. Even when in good condition, they irritated his skin with the adhesives he used to attach them.

Andy knew he would have to return to Mayo for further evaluation and checkups, but he had mixed feelings about his future treatments. Mardini had suggested that Andy might need as many as fifteen more reconstructive surgeries, including skin flaps and skin grafts, dental implants, and bone realignments. Even with all these procedures, Andy felt certain that in the end he would still appear disfigured.

Andy's first follow-up with Mardini came one month after his discharge from Mayo Clinic. The plastic surgeon wanted to see how well Andy's extensive reconstruction was holding up. In his initial exam, Mardini found Andy in good spirits and without complaints. He observed that Andy's surgical incisions were healing and had mostly closed, and that facial stretching exercises he had instructed Andy to do had slightly widened his mouth. Mardini had developed a schedule for future reconstruction: revisions of the upper lip, a dental prosthesis anchored into dental implants, and further work on Andy's facial soft tissues. Tissue expanders—inflatable plastic reservoirs used in reconstructive surgery to stretch overlying skin—were a possibility. Andy understood the work ahead and was willing to proceed.

During his visit, Andy also met again with Thomas Salinas, the prosthodontist who had created Andy's prosthetic nose. Salinas told Andy about the tooth implants he would receive in his next surgery. Looking over Andy's nose prosthesis, Salinas could see it was in ragged shape. Andy had been lax about cleaning it, which had to be done painstakingly with a toothbrush. After reiterating his instructions for cleaning the prosthesis and staying out of the sun as much as possible, Salinas sent him off to an appointment with psychologist Autumn Braddock.

Braddock wanted to check in on Andy's mood, his use of exposure therapy, and his search for mental health support in the vicinity of his home. "He notes being very social with his core group of friends," she wrote in his medical record. "He describes primarily staying at home and going over to other people's houses, and that he has been active in the community." That activity mostly amounted to shopping for groceries and buying home improvement supplies for his mother's house and tools at the hardware store.

Andy told Braddock that the exposure therapy had greatly reduced his aversion to his own face, although at one point he had felt a spike in his stress when examining his face closely in the mirror after removing his prosthetic nose. He became tearful and sad when talking about his facial injury but assured Braddock that he had not been thinking about or planning suicide. He also told Braddock that he did not know the combination to open the safe at home that held two firearms and so could not make any impulsive decisions to use them.

On June 5, 2007, Mardini successfully performed reconstructive surgery on Andy's upper lip, nasal passage, and mouth opening. Salinas also took impressions in Andy's mouth for future dental implants.

Over the next six years, Andy worked at rebuilding his life. He had wanted his old electrician apprentice job back in Casper, but there was no work for him there. This news disappointed him because he yearned to be where he was comfortable, around people who knew him, so he could begin to readjust. Instead, he found seasonal work as a cook and handyman at the Flying V Lodge, a hunting resort at the foot of the Black Hills in Newcastle. His employers, Larry and Twylla, had known Andy since his teenage years and gave him firm support.

Outside of his working hours, he frequently hunted nearby, often with Larry. "I'd get up, be out at 5:00 a.m., stay out hunting until 8:00, and then go to work," he remembered. After work he'd go hunting again, alone. Andy was not making much money working at the lodge and received no health insurance benefits, but the opportunity to hunt made the job worthwhile for him.

He also worked as a roustabout, or casual laborer, on an oil field, as well at a few other odd jobs. But he always found his way back to the lodge.

Being around other people was good for him and helped him to heal mentally and emotionally. Yet it also brought stress and anxiety. Every day his mind rattled with anxious worries. Where would his work take him? Who would be there? Would people be rude and obnoxious? Where would he eat lunch? This last question was a serious daily consideration. He often ate alone at work, because he did not want others to see him eat.

Andy largely believed in keeping to himself in these jobs, where he could avoid contact with other people. But sometimes people aggressively questioned him and tried to force him to explain his appearance. These incidents emotionally rocked him. "I'm the little scrawny guy—I'm not a big guy at all," he said. "I remember at a bar, this guy says to me, 'Who gave you the asshole where your face used to be?' I probably blacked out then because I got so angry."

The prosthetic nose was particularly a problem at work. To avoid damaging or discoloring it, Andy had to keep it away from oil, sun, and dirt. His work made this nearly impossible. "I dug ditches out in the oil field in the sun, so I was screwed," he said. He needed a new nose every few months, but he couldn't always afford the hundreds of dollars it cost to replace them. He sometimes painted the nose himself to keep it looking presentable and extend its life. "If I was just going to work, I wouldn't worry about it too much. But if I was going out with my friends, I painted it. I had figured out how to layer the paint to make it look more like my skin tone," he said. "You give it an undercoat of red and then work up to the skin tones." He was supposed to bake it in the oven to give the paint more permanence, but he usually skipped that step and simply painted it again when the color flaked off.

Andy also worried about whether coworkers would understand his speech and how he would manage to work outside in the cold, when his mouth tended to shrink up. "You're trying to plan all this stuff out inside your head. Like, 'I don't want to eat in front of these people. How can I get out of it? How do I not make a mess when I'm eating?' I'm trying so hard to do all these little things, and all that just builds up. It turns into anxiety," Andy said. He dreamed of showing up at a job site where he was just one of the guys, no one judged him or talked behind his back, and he earned respect for his skills.

Over the years, Andy focused his time and energy on people who could genuinely accept him, including his nephew, Lucas, and niece, Valerie, who were Ronald's children. They accepted Uncle Andy's appearance, and they had no idea he had ever looked different. On one occasion Andy was spending time with the children, who were jumping on a trampoline. One of Lucas's friends came over to join them. He looked at Andy and felt scared. "What's wrong with him?" the friend whispered. "There's nothing wrong with him," Lucas answered. "He just has a funny nose." The friend accepted that explanation and eventually grew accustomed to Andy's appearance.

But the thought that he might scare away children stuck in Andy's mind. He wondered if it would be better for him to spend less time with Ronald's kids, at least when they had friends over. He began asking in advance who else was coming to visit. "I didn't want to meet new people because of the way I was, just because I didn't want to have to tell a story and explain what happened," he says. "That was always an elephant in the room: 'What the hell happened to you?' I didn't want to talk about it because I felt ashamed—that's what it came down to."

Andy found solace in televised sports and sports websites. "Every single sport, it didn't matter," Andy says. He watched hockey, football, basketball, and even baseball, which was not his favorite. He bought subscriptions to sports networks and watched them all the time. When a game ended, he would move to online coverage and discussions. "That's how I used to deal with everything—just get lost in sports," he says. It was the only way he could feel or express emotions, whether happiness or anger. He did not know how else to access his inner self. But he refrained from fantasy sports because of the social aspect of those leagues. Andy could see himself growing more withdrawn and less communicative because of his disfigurement.

Five years after the treatment of his facial wounds at Mayo Clinic, Andy had received no formal counseling or psychiatric care for a long time. After his discharge from Mayo, Andy had promised himself that he would make sure his face was fixed by the time he reached thirty. What that exactly meant or would entail, he did not really know. But he was still no closer to that goal. "I just sat back and waited. My mom pushed me. 'You should call Dr. Mardini,' she said. I said, 'No, he's busy.'"

In truth, Andy was afraid to learn that nothing else could be done to improve his face. By not asking, he avoided the disappointment of hearing bad news. No communication meant he could keep alive in his mind the chance he could look close to normal someday.

∽

Mardini had been treating Andy for years now, and he felt frustrated that he could not bring Andy to a fuller recovery—or to where Andy wanted to be to find success and happiness in life. The plastic surgeon was dissatisfied with conventional techniques that could not achieve the outcomes Andy desired. "I couldn't see a way to make him look anywhere near normal, and that's extremely frustrating," Mardini said.

What about a face transplant? Andy's injury had occurred the year after the world's first such surgery. The procedure was so new that Mardini was unsure of the criteria to apply to prospective transplant patients, and he did not personally know any of the plastic surgeons who were performing transplants of this type.

The thought of Andy as a possible candidate came to mind, but there were implications to consider. Mardini reviewed Andy's photographs. "Not that bad, but when you say not that bad, what does it mean?" the plastic surgeon mused. "He doesn't have a nose. He's got this tiny mouth." Receiving a successful face transplant would solve some of these deficiencies for Andy. At the same time, performing a face transplant would destroy nearly all the original facial tissues and structures Andy had remaining. A failed transplant would be catastrophic.

Soon after Mardini arrived at Mayo in 2006, he and fellow plastic surgeon Steven Moran had begun talking with people in Mayo's transplant program about how to serve patients with amputations and significant facial injuries and disfigurement. The science of vascularized composite allotransplantation (VCA)—which involves transplantation of bone, nerve, muscle, and skin tissues as a unit, such as a face or hand, from deceased donors—was advancing rapidly.

The transplant center agreed certain plastic surgery patients could be helped, and Mayo's plastic surgeons began to examine what was possible. A big question was whether potential VCA patients, under consideration for receiving transplanted faces and hands, should be judged using criteria different from those for solid organ transplant patients who received hearts, livers, kidneys, and other internal organs. Mayo had established its programs for the transplant of those organs decades earlier and now had one of the largest, best, and most comprehensive centers in the country for solid organ transplantation.

The prospect of Mayo launching its own VCA program was still mostly talk at that time, however. "It was like something in the movies," Mardini said. "How cool. I don't want to say we weren't going to drive toward it, but it wasn't something that we were thinking about doing [every day]."

In 2011, Mardini experienced an unexpected and important change in his personal life. On a regular trip to Lebanon to visit family and friends, he met a young Lebanese woman, Rawan. They talked briefly at dinner. He was drawn to her beauty and kindness. "She was gracious and capable, talented and strong. I found her absolutely stunning," Mardini recalls.

Mardini returned to the United States, but Rawan remained in his thoughts. Six months later he was back in Lebanon. A resourceful man, he had managed to track down her number. Rawan took a call from him as she was eating in a restaurant with her mother. "I was very surprised," she said. Rawan agreed to see him again, and they spent hours talking over a view of the Mediterranean.

"I saw him as very calm and confident," Rawan said years later. "He was also grounded, and I realized from the first time I met him that he was special. He also just wanted to make sure that everybody around him was comfortable and happy. This characteristic really drew me to him." As a case in point, Rawan remembers a dinner date where her legs were being swarmed by mosquitoes as they were dining. Mardini immediately set off to fetch several kinds of relieving creams from the nearest pharmacy. "I knew this guy was a gem just from that," Rawan remembered.

A few weeks later, in the lobby of his hotel in Beirut, Mardini took Rawan's hand in his own and asked her to marry him. "Without hesitation, I said yes," she said. "Without thinking twice."

The previous year, Mardini had won an award from the American Society for Reconstructive Microsurgery, the year-long Godina Traveling Fellowship, a prestigious honor named after the innovative reconstructive microsurgeon and teacher Marko Godina. Godina's work in reconstructive surgery broke new ground in the field, but his career was cut short when he died in an auto accident at age forty-three.

The fellowship provided funding for Mardini to travel to world-renowned microsurgery centers and opened many doors—Mardini's credentials as a Godina Fellow encouraged fellow plastic surgeons to invite him to see their own visionary work. Mardini focused his fellowship year on facial transplant and the facial nerve, the study of which is closely linked to successful face transplantation. A personal highlight of some of these trips was seeing Rawan, who would meet up with him during his travels. In fact, much of their courtship was spent in hotel lobbies.

At the top of Mardini's to-do list was meeting patients who had undergone a face transplant. How could he consider bringing this procedure to his own patients without interviewing others who had been through it? He visited ten medical centers around the globe that had performed face transplants. He met Isabelle Dinoire, the world's first face transplant recipient, and three other patients. Mardini asked them about their concerns while undergoing the procedure, what it was like to have a face transplant, whether in hindsight they thought it was the best treatment they could have received, and if they would do it again. In addition, Mardini met with these patients' transplant surgeons and was impressed by their generosity and willingness to share their knowledge, experience, and insight. Mardini asked them about their techniques and experiences and listened to them discuss their patients. Given another chance with their patients, he inquired, would they do anything differently?

Mardini's goal was to make sure that Mayo's nascent VCA program for face and hand transplants would start at the highest level of advancement in the field at the current moment. He understood the importance of not repeating mistakes, and he was grateful that his peers were willing to share their experiences with him.

None of the patients Mardini met regretted their face transplants. They all adopted their new face as their own. Even the patients who did not emerge from their transplant with excellent functional or aesthetic results believed the transformation had restored their dignity and made them feel more human. They believed the transplant had dramatically improved their lives.

Mardini also learned that face transplant programs were most successful when one dynamic person led the surgical team. "There has to be that driving force, and if you look at every program, there is one person with that interest in helping the patient, who has the drive, ability, and leadership skills to conquer all the barriers, the ability to train and build a team, and the willingness to [work] with those patients for years to come," Mardini said.

During the fellowship, Mardini spent a few days with Laurent Lantieri, a French plastic surgeon who was one of the first to seriously consider face transplantation. Lantieri performed the world's third such operation and had since completed six others as well as a repeat transplant on one of his own patients. Mardini, who had met one of Lantieri's patients, asked the surgeon to speculate on the future of the face transplant procedure.

"He said this is the technology of today," Mardini remembered. "There isn't anything that's nearly as beneficial for patients right now." Other technologies on the horizon, such as improved immunosuppression and tissue engineering, might make transplants more successful or even supplant them in the future, but face transplant, Lantieri believed, was the best plastic surgery could now offer for patients who met the surgical criteria.

To help guide his own thoughts, Mardini created digital images that showed what Andy could look like after following two different paths: continued facial reconstruction or face transplant. He also investigated more mundane yet critical aspects of the matter, including how much a face transplant would cost and whether medical insurers would cover it.

"You're not comparing the cost of face transplant to doing nothing," Mardini said. "You're comparing it to doing fifteen other reconstructive surgeries, with each one having a hospitalization." He mapped out the comparison in a spreadsheet that

showed the steps required for each choice of treatment—length
of surgery, length of hospital stay, the patient's recovery time, and
more. "We calculated that, despite its formidable expense, the face
transplant would actually save money," based on the spreadsheet
data, Mardini says. "Financially, it's not a ridiculous route. It's a
reasonable route."

Mardini had learned a great deal about face transplants from
his travel fellowship, readings, and discussions with colleagues in
facial reconstruction. He also understood that some of his colleagues
might disagree with his pursuit of a face transplant for someone
like Andy—whose injuries did not put his life in jeopardy—
believing that the safest and most effective path was to use conventional reconstructive methods to bring their patients as close
to normal as possible while avoiding a perilous operation such as
face transplant and the risks involved in a lifetime of required
immunosuppression therapy.

On a visit to Mayo Clinic, Milomir Ninković, a skilled plastic
surgeon and friend of Mardini's, cautioned Mardini about facial
transplantation. He instead recommended further reconstructive
procedures, including nasal reconstruction, dental rehabilitation
with prosthetics, and lower lip reconstruction. Ninković asserted
he could reconstruct a nose and make it look acceptable after a few
operations. Mardini knew this was true, but he also knew that a
reconstructed nose would create facial scarring and require moving
tissue from the arm and rib cage. Furthermore, reconstruction
involved a trade-off, Mardini believed: accept mere improvement
and give up on a fully functional face of normal appearance. "You
find people who you respect, trust, and know they know what
they're saying. Even so, gathering multiple opinions from different
people, it was clear that face transplant was the way to go," Mardini
said. (Years later, when Ninković met Andy after his transplant,
Ninković admitted the results were much better than he
had expected.)

Nonetheless, there was a lot for Mardini and his colleagues to consider in Andy's case. It could be that Andy's psychological makeup did not make him a good candidate for face transplant. There were concerns about Andy's previous substance abuse and depression, and his resulting up-and-down outlook on life.

In addition, there were concerns about whether Andy had enough determination and social support to successfully handle the rigors of immunosuppressive therapy and tolerate its risks. After a transplant, recipients must follow a lifetime regimen of medications to suppress their bodies' natural immune responses and prevent rejection of the transplant. Long-term use of these medications can lead to kidney damage and failure, a complication that affects up to 20 percent of transplant recipients. In addition, immunosuppression regimens can spark the development of cancerous growths, weaken the patient's response to viral, bacterial, and fungal infections, and produce diabetes. No research suggested that VCA transplant patients would fare any differently.

Should Andy take those risks, or would they shorten his life unnecessarily? Salinas pointed out to Mardini that Andy could function without a face transplant. "After all, he could walk, he could talk, his speech was intelligible," he said. Salinas understood why Andy objected to his appearance, but was that enough of a reason to embark on the perilous journey of a face transplant?

# Chapter 6

# Decision

———

When Mardini began considering a face transplant for Andy, the procedure had existed for less than a decade, although exciting precursors of face transplant had been undertaken earlier than that.

A few prior cases had involved replants of the person's own facial tissue. In 1994, a nine-year-old Indian girl named Sandeep Kaur had had her face and scalp stripped from her head in an accident with a threshing machine. With remarkable presence of mind, the girl's mother gathered the ripped flesh in a plastic bag and set off on a broken-down moped for the nearest hospital. The journey took three and a half hours. By chance, a skilled microsurgeon, Abraham Thomas, was on duty that day at Christian Medical College and Hospital in Ludhiana, in northwest India.

Thomas regarded the salvaged face and scalp as a gift because it was the girl's own facial tissue. At the time, the only other possibility would be to retrieve skin grafts from elsewhere on Sandeep's body to repair her extensive injuries. But this surely would result in a profoundly disfigured face. Skin from other places on the body has texture and coloration different from facial skin and makes for poor-looking reconstructed mouths and noses.

Sandeep's rescued facial tissue offered the best approach. It was a magical moment during the reattachment when Thomas began suturing Sandeep's arteries and saw the skin of the facial flesh turn pink, signaling the return of circulating blood to the tissue. What amounted to a face replant proved surprisingly successful. Despite scarring and damage to her facial muscles, the girl recovered and resumed her life, beginning training as a nurse eleven years after the accident. An American team at Massachusetts General Hospital performed a similar replant in 2002 to treat a factory worker whose hair and face had been torn off by a conveyor belt.

These treatments, though not technically transplants, raised a tantalizing question: was transplanting a donor's face to a patient within the realm of possibility?

During the twentieth century, solid organ transplants from deceased donors had become possible as medicine tamed the human immune system with steadily improving reliability. Joseph Murray, who later shared a Nobel Prize for his transplant work, performed the first solid organ transplant, a kidney from an identical twin donor, in 1954. Following this surgery, which did not require immunosuppression because of the genetic match between the twins, the steroid prednisone soon became one of the immunosuppression drugs of choice to prevent organ rejection after such procedures. Cyclosporine, a fungal derivative that in 1976 was found to greatly dampen immune response, became a later foundation of immunosuppressive treatments despite its potential toxicity and side effects. Livers, hearts, and other organs joined the list of transplantable body parts. Later, in the 1990s, a more effective immunosuppressive drug, tacrolimus, would largely supplant cyclosporine.

In 1987, British plastic surgeon James Frame recalled years later, he and his colleague Roy Saunders were on the verge of performing a face transplant on a patient with an invasive squamous cell carcinoma, but the patient withdrew consent on the morning of the scheduled operation. Had the surgeons been able to perform this procedure, nearly twenty years before the next attempt, the history of face transplant would be much different today.

In 1991, the first medical conference focusing on vascularized composite allotransplantation (VCA) procedures—primarily face and hand transplants—took place in Washington, D.C. Hand transplants, conceptually related to face transplants because both involve the transplant of bone, muscle, skin, and circulatory and nerve tissue, were the first to have success.

Australian surgeon Earl Owen and French surgeon Jean-Michel Dubernard carried out the first successful hand transplant in 1998 in Lyon, France. The patient, who had lost his hand in an accident eleven years earlier, received his transplanted hand from a deceased donor. Expecting that face transplants were soon to follow, American surgeon John Barker noted that in many respects "a face is just like a hand." The similarity of the techniques used in transplanting hands and faces, or so it was speculated, would bring about successful surgeries involving these bundles of tissue types. Unfortunately, the hand recipient in the French transplant stopped adhering to his immunosuppression therapy and subsequently asked to have the transplanted hand amputated, highlighting the fact that transplantation is not for everyone. In 1999, a surgical team at the University of Louisville carried out the world's second and longest-surviving hand transplant. In doing so, it used immunosuppression drug combinations that were already being used in solid organ transplant recipients.

By the end of the twentieth century, vascularized composite allotransplantation of faces edged into the realm of possibility. In

2002, British plastic surgeon Peter Butler, who had been studying and rehearsing face transplant techniques for years, declared to a medical conference audience that the expertise now existed to perform face transplants. But five years later, there had been no face transplants in the United Kingdom; Butler's work had been handicapped by the public perception that "this is the stuff of Gothic horror, grave robbers, and Victorian freaks shows," as journalist Simon Hattenstone wrote.

Beyond those unattractive associations, still needing resolution were concerns about the value of face transplants versus the risks for patients. The goal in traditional organ transplantation was clear—to replace a failed organ and prolong the life of the patient. The goal for the transplant of other body parts, faces and hands among them, was less clear. Was the main aim cosmetic, functional, or psychological?

In the case of face transplants, a consensus slowly formed that though these were not lifesaving procedures, they could greatly improve patients' quality of life, including the ability to eat, blink, talk, and make facial expressions. It could also improve their psychological well-being and ability to reintegrate into society. "After the other doctors leave," the surgeon Bohdan Pomahac told *The New Yorker* in a discussion of such transplants, "we're the ones who try to help the patient be functional and live a normal life." Face transplants are not lifesaving, but they are life-giving.

The challenge of face and hand transplants was in the proper planning and execution of the procedures. To achieve good functional and aesthetic outcomes, the nerves of the donor had to be connected properly to the nerves of the recipient, the bones had to be precisely aligned, and the muscles had to be joined together in a way that allowed for unencumbered movement.

Maria Siemionow, a surgeon at Cleveland Clinic, began pondering the possibility of face transplants in the 1980s while treating burn patients in Mexico. There were surgical procedures that helped children with badly burned hands, she knew—so why not for patients with injured faces? She earned approval from Cleveland Clinic to perform face transplants in 2004. The Polish-trained plastic surgeon tested scores of techniques, including suturing patterns for nerves and blood vessels and new immunosuppressive approaches. Early on, she succeeded in transplanting new faces to laboratory rats. Although some of her colleagues discouraged her work as a waste of time with little applicability to patients, she identified human candidates for her face transplant program.

Meanwhile, surgical teams from China, Spain, the United States, and France competed to perform the first face transplant on a human patient. The British medical journal *The Lancet* offered an article to its readers in 2002 speculating on the future of the yet-untried procedure. Soon after, in 2003, following an eight-month study, the Royal College of Surgeons discouraged the pursuit of face transplants. It cited the potential for long-term pharmacological effects and tissue rejection if immunosuppressive medications did not work as well for face transplant recipients as they did for solid organ recipients, and the unknown psychological effects on patients' and donors' families.

The first team to perform a face transplant never publicly announced its intention to enter the field. In 2005, Isabelle Dinoire awoke after an overdose of sleeping pills and discovered that her pet Labrador retriever had severely mauled her face, presumably while trying to wake her. Her image in the mirror was terrifying and scarcely human, she said. Her mouth was torn apart, with teeth and gums exposed. After conventional reconstructive treatment that left her visibly disfigured, she dreaded leaving home and did so only if she wore a surgical mask. Scar tissue was forming in a web, making her appearance even worse. Dinoire was depressed and isolated, and her physicians worried that her condition, left unimproved, would worsen her mental state and alcohol dependency and prompt more suicidal impulses. The social damage that facial disfigurement wrought in Dinoire's case and others figured prominently in the arguments of face transplant advocates.

After much deliberation, craniofacial surgeons at Centre Hospitalier Universitaire d'Amiens, led by Bernard Devauchelle, embarked on a face transplant for Dinoire on November 27, 2005. They worked in cooperation with Dubernard in Lyon, who had performed the first successful hand transplant. Dubernard's team took charge of obtaining governmental and hospital approvals, bringing together the surgical team, and supervising the postoperative immunosuppression.

The thirty-eight-year-old Dinoire's transplant involved the nose, chin, and mouth from a donor—soft tissue only, a partial face transplant. She eventually regained enough function to speak, smile, drink from a glass, and smoke (a habit plastic surgeons strongly discouraged for such patients). The operation had occurred without any preliminary public discussion, publicity, or debate. When Dinoire's face transplant became known, it created an explosion of international interest. "A door to the future is opening," Dinoire said in a public statement. Despite some immunosuppressant-related complications and unwanted media attention, it appeared that the surgery had benefited Dinoire. Dinoire died in 2016 of lung cancer possibly related to immunosuppressant therapy.

Some critics of the procedure wondered whether face transplants would evolve into merely a cosmetic treatment for the rich. Nevertheless, the heights of the French achievement seemed so impressive that Devauchelle—no paragon of modesty—told reporters his professional guide and hero was not another surgeon. Instead, he had looked to the Everest-conquering mountaineer Sir Edmund Hillary for his inspiration. Most important to the face transplant debate, the operation offered proof that the procedure could be done.

A Chinese team performed the world's second face transplant in 2006. The patient was a thirty-year-old man, Li Guoxing, the victim of a mauling by a bear. Li survived only two years after his operation because on his own initiative he replaced his immuno-suppression medication with unapproved herbal remedies. Some surgeons questioned whether Li had received adequate psychological screening before the transplant.

These early face transplants signaled an important advance in possibilities for people with debilitating facial injuries and defor-mities. Later face transplants drew on previous efforts. From the soft tissue transplant that Dinoire received in 2005, the procedure grew to include bones and an increasing number of functional units, eventually including such major facial bone structures as the upper jaw, lower jaw, bones forming the eye orbits, and bones that form the cheek arches. Still, for several years all face transplants were partial transplants. Nobody had yet performed a full-face transplant that included tissues all the way up to the hairline.

In late 2008, however, Siemionow of the Cleveland Clinic came close. Siemionow's patient was forty-five-year-old Connie Culp, who had been shot in the face by her husband, leaving her unable to breathe or eat without assistance. In an operation that took twenty-three hours, she received the inside tissues of a donor's mouth, the upper and lower jaws, and the nose, along with 80 percent of the facial skin. "Don't judge people who don't look the same as you do," Culp told reporters when she went public about her transplant, "because you never know. One day it might be all taken away." She made a guest appearance on *Oprah* and publicly met and thanked her donor's family—a first.

Two years later, a Spanish team performed the first full-face transplant, a procedure successfully repeated in 2011 at Brigham and Women's Hospital in Boston. Because many of these involved additions of bone that restored the normal contours of the face, the results of full-face transplants appeared cosmetically more pleasing than earlier attempts. Patients sometimes said they felt the return of partial sensation in their faces three months after the operation, with full sensation arriving eight to twelve months after the transplant. Many previous face transplants had achieved only spotty or incomplete sensation. Results related to motor function of the face muscles, an essential aspect of face transplantation, were extremely variable.

Despite some poor cosmetic results, "the aesthetic outcomes after face transplantation are generally acceptable and, in some cases, even exceed the expectations," declared Maria Siemionow in the *Journal of Materials Science*. Nearly all patients endured some tissue rejection, major or minor. Most said they were happy with their transplants. Some even returned to work and fully rejoined their old social circles. "In the second decade, we will make face transplantation safer and applicable to the broader population of severely disfigured patient[s] worldwide," Siemionow predicted.

Meanwhile, the Armed Forces Institute of Regenerative Medicine, a consortium of military and private institutions located in Fort Detrick, Maryland, became a financial supporter of face transplant research and three surgeries at Cleveland Clinic. The organization grew from efforts to improve treatment for the hundreds of U.S. military veterans who returned injured from the Iraq War and other conflicts. The U.S. Department of Defense funded face transplants performed by the team of Bohdan Pomahac and Julian Pribaz at Brigham and Women's Hospital in Boston.

At the Chauvet Workgroup, an international conference in 2014 led by Mayo psychiatrist Sheila Jowsey-Gregoire and others, a group of people involved in transplantation—surgeons, psychiatrists, and directors of transplant programs—met to discuss approaches to evaluating hand transplant candidates, and to monitor the recovery and adjustment of patients after their surgeries. Mardini attended the conference and encouraged that the face be included. In the nine years following the first face transplant in 2005, some three dozen patients had received new faces or partial faces. Five died from a variety of causes: surgical complications, refusal or inability to take their immunosuppressive medications properly, suicide, or the recurrence of previously treated cancers.

To the surprise of critics who challenged the ethics of the procedure based on its absence of lifesaving potential, face transplant had gained momentum, producing good outcomes for patients. Only four face transplants had been performed in the world between 2005 and 2008, but twenty-seven partial- and full-face surgeries followed between 2009 and 2013.

Although most programs did not clearly disclose the cost of the face transplants they performed, the amount was usually comparable to that of other highly complicated procedures, such as combined heart and lung transplantations.

Mardini's colleagues often talk about his fondness for close collaboration and the high respect he holds for the opinions of others, both colleagues and patients. When a patient's case does not progress as expected, he refuses to simply move on. "He will bring that case up, not once, not twice, but dozens of times to brainstorm with the team what else we can do, what we are missing, how we can do things differently," says Mayo neurologist Beth Robertson, a facial nerve expert and a key member of Mardini's facial reanimation team. She recalls receiving many phone calls at night from Mardini to discuss alternative procedures and new treatments for patients both of them were treating. She believes he is always thinking of people who can provide new ideas, a habit he developed during his five-year experience in Taiwan. "He works with input from surgeons worldwide. He will go and follow and watch them, train with them, and ask them questions until he gets what he thinks is the very best possible surgical approach for that specific patient," Robertson says, "and that's incredible."

In 2006 and 2007, with Andy Sandness's case still fresh in his mind, Mardini had begun discussing with Mayo colleagues the possibility of launching a hand and face transplant effort. The head of the institution's well-established transplant center, transplant cardiologist Brooks Edwards, listened to Mardini with interest. "I admired his willingness to entertain this wild idea," Mardini said of Edwards. It would have been easy to take a safe and conservative approach to the guidance of an institution-wide reconstructive transplant center, but Edwards was a driver and innovator. He was supportive, "just the right amount," Mardini says. "He was not in your face—he just helped and backed us up and was there when needed." Edwards offered mentoring, advice, and more while guiding the effort through Mayo's institutional committees and the processes of LifeSource, the Upper Midwest's organ procurement organization.

Edwards suggested Mardini team with Hatem Amer, a brilliant and dedicated transplant nephrologist who was working with Mayo's kidney and pancreas transplant patients. In Amer, Edwards saw a young yet experienced innovator and hoped he would agree to become the medical director of Mayo's hand and face transplant program. (Amer would soon receive Mayo's Karis Award for representing the institution's values to the fullest degree.)

"Getting a transplant is a new lease on life, and for me [face transplant] was a very interesting area to go into, and I like the science behind it as well," said Amer. He soon immersed himself in the VCA field by attending conferences, going to VCA meetings, and meeting many hand and face transplant surgeons and other specialists involved in the care of VCA patients. As the program's medical director, Amer could look after the medical and immunosuppressive needs of face transplant patients. Mardini and Moran would serve as surgical directors of the new program—Mardini would take charge of face transplants and Moran would lead hand transplants.

Amer had a reputation for being focused and methodical. "He's not going to make a mistake in anything he does," Mardini says. "This is probably how he is with everything. He went into it full force." Before becoming medical director of the program, Amer "had nothing to do with hand surgery. He had nothing to do with craniofacial surgery." Yet Amer learned the details of every face and hand transplant attempted to date. He would become a leader and critical team member in the development of the program and in the treatment of Andy Sandness.

Pursuing face transplants is a complex endeavor. A successful outcome vastly improves the patient's life, but an unsuccessful surgery can lead to the patient's premature death. Furthermore, face transplants are complicated surgeries that take dozens of hours and involve the removal of remaining structural parts of the face. A transplant that goes wrong could leave the patient more seriously disfigured than before, possibly with no face at all. In such a disastrous outcome, surgeons would have to transplant tissue from other parts of the body—likely abdominal tissue or the latissimus muscle of the back—just to cover the open wound. Or the patient could end up with a face that does not move or function properly. Surgeons must be mindful of the possibility of running into that horrific situation, and they must be prepared for it. Even if a face transplant initially goes well, patients have a real risk of encountering subsequent problems such as tissue rejection, kidney failure, skin and other types of cancers, and other side effects from immunosuppressive treatment.

Mardini quickly learned virtually everything there was to know about the field of face transplantation. Along with Amer, Edwards, administrator Lori Ewoldt, and others, Mardini used his expertise to present to several Mayo committees, starting with those within the transplant center focusing on ethics and clinical practice. The team later presented their plans to other institutional bodies. To Mayo's Clinical Practice Committee, the group delivered a proposal for a VCA transplant program, which the committee approved in due course. Meanwhile, Mardini mentioned his face transplant aspirations to John Noseworthy, then chief executive officer of Mayo Clinic. "I could see the twinkle in his eye," Noseworthy remembered, "his belief that if face transplants are going to help patients, Mayo Clinic should do this and do it well."

Mayo wanted to run its VCA transplant program well, even if it differed from other models in the United States. Most such programs were organized as research endeavors, in part because face and hand transplantations were considered experimental. In addition, funding for research programs was available from the Department of Defense.

But Mayo's planners determined that the number of successful VCA transplants that had already taken place, along with the many commonplace techniques that these transplants combined, made the procedures no longer experimental. As long as standard immunosuppressive therapies were used, the program could be run as a clinical endeavor. VCA patients were not really candidates for experimental immunosuppressive treatments, given their small numbers and the risks involved should the grafts fail. The leadership of Mayo's Institutional Review Board noted that Mardini and his VCA colleagues were welcome to submit studies of specific aspects of VCA transplantation. Looking back, it now appears that Mayo's approach, of setting up the program as a clinical program, not a research program, brought advantages. Among them—crucially important to patients—was that a clinical procedure allowed for the possibility of medical insurance coverage over the long term, while a research procedure might not. It also allowed the Mayo VCA program to proceed without the pressure to enroll a certain number of subjects within a given study period, which meant that the program could focus on identifying the best path for each patient, whether that was conventional treatment or VCA transplantation.

At the time Mayo was laying the groundwork for its vascularized composite allotransplantation program for hand and face transplants, the science behind VCA was changing rapidly. There was as yet no guidance or oversight from any health authority or government agency on starting a VCA program. Mayo had to set up its own procedures and establish its own path forward, and it would not enter this sphere of medicine cavalierly.

Mayo set out to investigate how VCA protocols and screening might be similar to or different from solid organ transplant protocols and screening. The decision was made that the Mayo VCA programs would follow the same regulations as solid organ transplant programs, including multidisciplinary selection conferences and mandated communication with transplant candidates about their status. The disciplines involved would include those usually seen in other solid organ transplant programs, such as registered nurses certified as transplant coordinators, pharmacists, dietitians, clinical transplant social workers, and transplant financial counselors. Additional specialists deemed important to VCA included plastic surgeons, who were brought on for joint appointments in 2010, as well as physical and occupational therapists and clinical ethicists.

Lori Ewoldt, who in her role as transplant center administrator had experience in all administrative aspects of solid organ transplants and bone marrow transplants, took on many of the new VCA program challenges. "She has that really caring quality of understanding people and understanding patients," Mardini said. An Iowa native, Ewoldt has spent her entire career at Mayo and worked for years in a variety of nursing positions before handling operations in the transplant center.

Getting VCA transplants approved at Mayo was a huge task. Many staff members familiar with the needs of transplant patients came forward to participate in the new effort. Their goal was to create a high level of caring, true to Mayo's principles. Ultimately, the core VCA team at Mayo included about fifty people.

The Mayo VCA transplant team sent members to VCA centers in Kentucky and France to tour their facilities and meet hand and face transplant team members and their patients. They learned about the benefits and drawbacks of VCA procedures, different outcome possibilities, and the results of various allotransplants. Those visits brought valuable information on the distinctive needs of amputees and facial disfigurement patients, both before and after transplants. "We understood that the psychiatric component is going to be extremely critical," said Hatem Amer. "We do mental health checks by a transplant psychiatrist on all the transplant recipients when they go through their evaluation."

The psychiatric demands on traditional solid organ recipients and VCA recipients are different. Mayo psychiatrist Sheila Jowsey-Gregoire, despite extensive experience in working with solid organ recipients, had to establish new tools to evaluate VCA transplant candidates. "It would be wonderful if we could just give a patient a computerized test and they passed," she said. "But patients who come for transplant are typically very motivated for transplant, so, like any good job applicant, they'll be looking to present themselves in the best way to move forward with the transplant"—a reflection not of any intent to deceive but of their desire to receive access to the treatment they perceived as having the greatest benefit.

Jowsey-Gregoire instead found a different way to assess candidates for face transplant surgery. She focused on the reality of their lives, not the best version of themselves they could present. They were otherwise healthy people who had to weigh the pros and cons of the surgery and lifelong immunosuppression. Jowsey-Gregoire and her psychiatric colleagues working in VCA programs around the world developed psychological evaluations that took measure of that decision-making capability. She tried to find ways to capture the ten qualities that the American psychiatrist Dennis S. Charney, an expert in neurobiology, had set forth as essential for living through difficult experiences: optimism, problem-solving, flexibility, having a support network, having a resilient role model, using exercise as a way to cope, helping others, accepting things for what they are, having faith, and cultivating a sense of humor.

Jowsey-Gregoire has those essential qualities memorized and likes to recite them. Her work has since influenced the evaluation of VCA patients in many programs. Together with Palmina Petruzzo, Martin Kumnig, and Emmanuel Morelon, she established the international Chauvet Workgroup for the Psychosocial Aspects of VCA.

"To be able to communicate, to be able to gesture, to be able to hold somebody's hand, to be able to have a face that doesn't stand out in a way that's distracting—all of those things are very important," Jowsey-Gregoire said.

Mardini's intent was not simply to perform a face transplant on Andy; it was to provide the right treatment for him. "You have to think really hard if the patient would benefit from it," he said. "If the patient is willing to do it, and if you actually have enough of a passion and love for that patient that you want to go through that journey with them. It's a lifelong journey." Mardini double- and triple-checked his thoughts on Andy's candidacy for the procedure. Few patients, he knew, had the requisite psychological strength, courage, and willingness.

Even as the possibility of performing face transplants at Mayo approached reality, Mardini continued to look at conventional reconstructive surgeries for Andy. If the latter proved to be the best course for Andy, Mardini wanted to have the future course of reconstruction mapped out. Mardini believed there were two reasons for outlining Andy's possible path with conventional reconstructive techniques. It would allow for a realistic understanding of the likely functional and aesthetic outcome of traditional treatment; it would also enable Mardini to give medical insurance companies a complete picture of the comparative benefits and risks of reconstruction versus face transplantation when the time came to determine coverage.

If Andy's face was to be traditionally reconstructed, Mardini could take a flap from Andy's arm to reconstruct the inner lining of the nose. Then he could use some of Andy's extant lower lip to add to the inadequate upper lip, and completely replace the lower lip with a functional, innervated gracilis muscle from the inside of his thigh. Mardini would have to operate in multiple stages to debulk the reconstructed nose and make it look thin and refined, and Andy would be left with open areas on his forehead, from which grafts would serve as the outside of the nose, that would eventually heal and create scar tissue. A third phase would be dental rehabilitation, aligning the upper bone of the jaw with the lower bone before adding tooth implants and widening the opening of the mouth. From start to finish, this series of reconstructive surgeries would take a year or two.

When Mardini brought up Andy's case with his colleagues at Mayo and elsewhere, he asked them about treatments for central facial deformities like Andy's. The general verdict: a surgeon can work on these patients for years using conventional reconstructive surgery, but in the end, a central facial deformity remains. The surgeries can help them look a little better and can restore some function to their faces, yet they will still appear disfigured. The sheer number of operations needed in the years ahead, Mardini realized, along with Andy's sincere quest to look and function the way most people do—the fervent desire of most patients in his situation—made continued facial reconstruction an unsatisfying choice.

Mardini also considered the possibility of other emerging treatments. Advances in tolerance induction—new techniques to build a person's tolerance for cells from other bodies without the need for the harsh immune-suppressing drugs currently in use—might be one avenue. If, for example, a safe and reliable means of inducing tolerance to organs obtained from a deceased donor could be achieved, then the risk-benefit ratio for VCA transplant would shift in favor of performing transplants of smaller and smaller functional and aesthetic units.

Another possibility might be tissue engineering, an emerging technology that creates a living frame, or matrix, for a body part that needs replacement, such as the nose. A matrix embedded with stem cells and substances that stimulate cell growth could theoretically allow tissue from Andy's own body to grow into a structure that would look and function like a nose. Although tissue engineering was becoming more sophisticated and advanced, the technology was still limited and was not yet in clinical use. In addition, body parts more complex than the nose, such as cheeks and jaws, are composed of a multitude of separate structures that typically function in concert, making engineered versions even further from reality for many transplant patients.

Facial prosthetics, while offering Andy additional possibilities, could only enhance appearance, not offer function. No prosthetic then on the horizon would have allowed a patient like Andy to smile or would provide an eating passageway. Prosthetics also require frequent cleaning and changing.

It seemed that none of these treatments could yet match the feeling and function provided by successful transplants. "Maybe they will fifty years from now," Mardini says. They are technologies of the future, whereas face transplant was a treatment of the moment.

What makes someone a good candidate for a face transplant? Medically, of course, they must have an anatomic defect for which face transplant is an appropriate treatment. In addition, they must have psychosocial strength and stability, because a face transplant is a long and arduous ordeal. They must have courage and the willingness to undergo the difficult surgery and recovery. They must also have realistic expectations of the outcome of the face transplant. And they must be comfortable with some uncertainty. Because of the short time face transplants have been used as a treatment, nobody knows how long the transplanted tissues will last.

Finally, to afford the best chances for a successful outcome, both patient and surgeon must be comfortable having a long-term professional relationship based on mutual trust. A highly complex operation such as a face transplant requires a close, long, and demanding relationship between transplant team and patient— connections longer and deeper than those shared for most other kinds of treatment. "It's a lifelong journey," says Mardini.

After exploring the pros and cons of face transplant for Andy from many different angles, Mardini finally made his decision based on his extensive background, training, and experience in facial reconstruction, craniofacial surgery, facial nerve surgery, and reconstructive microsurgery. Before Mardini came to Mayo Clinic, people had idly but encouragingly told him he had the skills, passion, talents, and team-building skills to do a face transplant. "It sounded really cool," Mardini remembers, "but it really didn't mean much" to him then. When Andy first arrived at Mayo after his suicide attempt three months after Mardini joined the Mayo staff, the world's first face transplant had been done only a year before. The procedure had not yet caught Mardini's serious attention. Some five years later, he believed he could make one happen. And Andy seemed to meet the criteria now formulating in Mardini's mind.

Since Andy's treatment and reconstruction from his gunshot wound in 2006, Mardini had seen his patient somewhat irregularly over the following years. Andy had been reluctant to call Mardini, worried that he would be bothering the busy physician. Mardini placed a phone call to Andy in Wyoming in the spring of 2012. "I said, 'Look, can you come out and visit? Because I have colleagues around the world who have performed face transplants on patients with similar deformities to yours. I want you to know that this is maybe a possibility,'" Mardini said.

Shortly thereafter, Andy and Rhonda met Mardini and members of his team in Rochester. The plastic surgeon told them that Mayo was going to start a face transplant program. Mardini went on to suggest that he and Andy, whom the plastic surgeon considered a strong candidate for the procedure, might work together to explore the possibilities.

Andy felt ecstatic; he asked how soon he could get the transplant. "I wanted to jump right in," he remembered in an interview nearly a decade later. Even so, Mardini believed he had to temper his patient's excitement. At that point, only about thirty face transplants had been performed in the world—and only a few in the United States. There were risks, a long period of recovery, and a regimen of immunosuppressant drugs that Andy would have to take for the rest of his life, wherever he lived and whatever his life circumstances. In other words, the treatment was laden with the real possibility of complications over time.

Mardini wanted Andy to slow down and make a fully informed decision about his own future. The looming choice was huge. Andy would go from being a perfectly healthy (although disfigured) person to someone who—because of the harmful effects of immunosuppression therapy after surgery—would be involved with doctors and taking medicine for the rest of his life. There was a risk Andy could die during the transplant operation. "I want you to do your own research. Use Google," Mardini said, countering the advice of some physicians who caution patients against seeking medical information on the internet. "Learn as much as you can about what the procedure entails and what's been done so far." He offered to connect Andy with patients who had undergone the procedure.

"It was a little surreal," Mardini observed. "You're having a discussion that you never had before with a patient and that no one you ever trained with had with their patients." Many others on the transplant team, including Amer and Mayo's psychiatrists, would also have to weigh in.

Different but equally profound thoughts ran through Andy's mind. "When you look like I looked and you function like I functioned," he later said, "every little bit of hope that you have, you just jump on it." He fervently hoped a face transplant would bring him back to normal. What he most yearned for was normal function, not looks. He wanted everything he no longer had: a working nose, full-sized mouth, lips, and teeth. He dreamed of swimming, eating without embarrassment, and kissing. After the ordeal of his suicide attempt and the reconstruction of his face, Andy hoped for a second chance.

"We brought it to his attention. Then it revved up his engines," Mardini said. "We had a collaborative drive to getting this done rather than one person pushing much more than another. When he realized [this possibility] was out there, when he started thinking he [was] a potential candidate, when he started understanding more about it and seeing that this [was] a way to becoming more 'normal,' he started pushing a lot harder."

That conversation changed everything. It sparked Andy's hope. Up to that time, Andy always told Mardini in their conversations that he was doing fine. Indeed, Andy believed he was doing fine—did he have a choice? But the face transplant conversation poured accelerant on Andy's dreams for his future and his relationship with Mardini. "It got more intense," Mardini remembered.

Mardini did not want Andy's expectations to run wild. "Think very hard about this," he urged Andy. While Andy was weighing the decision he had to make, Laurent Lantieri—the surgeon who had already performed multiple face transplants—came to Mayo

Clinic for a conference Mardini hosted on reconstructive micro-surgery, one of sixty leading surgeons who attended. Mardini asked Lantieri if he would meet Andy and give his advice on this case. Lantieri obliged. Mardini set up a meeting at which several other prominent surgeons were present. Andy felt honored and appreciative to have the chance to hear the opinions of Lantieri and this group of world leaders in craniofacial reconstruction. If it could carry him one step closer to a successful treatment, Andy was willing.

In a vacant lecture hall alongside the lab where Mardini was supervising cadaver studies that were part of the conference, Lantieri met Andy and his mother. He questioned Andy on his lifestyle—whether and what he smoked, how much he drank, what he did when he socialized with others. "I told him the truth on everything," Andy says. "He sat back and he started analyzing in his head." Lantieri told Andy, "Yes, you're a candidate.'" This was reassuring to Mardini, and Rhonda gasped with excitement and relief. Andy told his mother to calm down. "They haven't said it's going to happen," he reminded her.

Lantieri told Mardini that if it were his decision, he would perform a face transplant on Andy. At this time Andy and his mom were under lots of stress from their long drive to Mayo, the ava-lanche of information they had received, and the big decision ahead. A click of resolve sounded in Andy's mind. "I thought, 'We've got to do this,'" he recalls.

Andy and Rhonda returned to Wyoming after meeting Lantieri. For months after that they heard nothing from Mardini. Rhonda urged Andy to check in with the doctor via email. Andy declined, knowing how busy Mardini always was. At last they heard again from Mardini in November 2012. In the intervening months, there had been a happy event for Mardini—he and Rawan had married and taken a honeymoon in the Maldives. Now they were back in

Rochester. In the years ahead, the Mardinis would go on to create a home together in Rochester and raise four children.

Everything was moving ahead with the face transplant evaluation, the surgeon assured Andy. Mardini explained that launching the new transplant program was a long process. He suggested that Andy and Rhonda return to Mayo in a few months for more discussions about what a transplant would demand of Andy and his family. In addition, Andy received the news that Mayo might be willing to cover the costs of his treatment as a charity case if he met the criteria.

Andy heard from Mardini and other Mayo physicians about the possibility of tissue rejection in a face transplant, which would be a serious complication. If a patient's immune system rejects a transplanted internal organ, surgeons can sometimes remove the rejected organ and perform a repeat transplant, with the patient being not much worse off than before the treatment. Although repeat face transplants are possible, they require a waiting period for an appropriate donor. Transplanting a face requires cutting and often removing the base structures of the patient's head—including bones, nerves, and blood vessels—and undoing the transplant would leave the patient with a dire lack of essential components of the face, with a high likelihood of death.

Mardini realized there was nothing good about the exit strategy from an unsuccessful face transplant. In Andy's case, in which the upper and lower jaws along with all the overlying facial structures would be transplanted, the proper preparation of Andy's face to receive that much tissue required the removal of all his original facial structures except the eyeballs, the back of the maxillary sinuses, the back of the throat, the tongue, and such critical blood vessels of the neck as the carotid artery and the internal jugular veins. With so much of his other facial tissues gone, there would be little opportunity for a second chance in the event of a failed transplant.

In addition, Hatem Amer described possible side effects of the immunosuppressive medications Andy would have to take for life—the development of diabetes, renal disease, and infection among them—and how he would have to avoid certain foods such as sushi, which might open the door to infection, and grapefruit, which could affect his body's metabolization of some medications. Opportunistic infectious agents like cytomegalovirus, common and usually harmless in most people but possibly fatal in those with weakened immune systems, along with Epstein-Barr virus, could also take root because of the patient's immunosuppressed state. The odds of skin cancer increase as well, which would require Andy to take extra precautions in his exposure to the sun—he would have to use sunscreen and wear a hat whenever possible. Yet immunosuppression was mandatory. Andy wondered whether he could stick to the intensive medication regimen. "I'm one of those people that hate being told what not to do or what to do," Andy says. "I always think I can do whatever I want. That's the mentality I have. I'm going to prove you wrong—that I can do it." Such choices could prove fatal after a face transplant.

"I had to step back from the stubborn self," Andy says, "if I was going to go through with this surgery." Back in Wyoming, he questioned his suitability for a face transplant. Until his suicide attempt in 2006, he had been healthy all his life. No broken bones, barely even the need for Tylenol to relieve headaches. The possibility of experiencing side effects from the immunosuppressive drugs or eating something that messed up his medications rattled him. "More than anything, I was scared of the medicine and not the surgery," he said.

Beyond Andy's personal attitudes, Mayo had to entertain ethical considerations regarding his treatment. The first consideration, at play with any patient, was informed consent. "Does the patient truly understand not only the potential benefit, which in this case is rather dramatic?" said Michael Bannon, a Mayo surgeon

and bioethicist who at the time chaired Mayo Clinic's ethics committee. "Does he know for sure the risks involved and, indeed, the
novelty of the procedure and the fact that we haven't done
this before?"

To make a truly reasoned decision, Andy had to balance the
risk of the unknown and possible complications against the potential
benefits. Even after a face transplant that succeeded surgically, did
Andy understand that the facial functions he desperately sought
might not materialize, at least not in all the ways he hoped? Did
he comprehend that the surgery might leave him with only partial
sensation in his face and less than full control of his facial muscles?

The medical staff goes through a similar weighing of risks and
benefits. A face transplant is not a lifesaving operation in the same
sense that a heart transplant is, and it may shorten the patient's life
because of the stresses and dangers of the immunosuppression
therapy. The procedure is potentially life-giving and life-enhancing,
however, as transplant surgeons have pointed out. And, despite
good intentions, some transplant patients neglect to take their
medications when they should.

Are the benefits and improvements to the patient's quality of
life sufficient to justify the risk? Over a three-month period, Mardini
and his colleagues repeatedly discussed the procedure and this
question. This extended discussion allowed all the important considerations to sink in, and it made space for the perspectives of
many people at Mayo, from many different medical disciplines, to
be fully reviewed. For Mardini, weighing the potential benefits to
Andy against the real risks forced him to deepen his understanding
of all aspects of face transplantation, and the challenge and thrill
of the procedure enthralled him. He collected advice and opinions
from experts in the fields of psychiatry, plastic surgery, ethics,
and others.

Among the ethical considerations was how Mayo would inform
the public of an imminent face transplant, or the completion of

one. At other medical centers, the names of patients who had undergone face transplants were sometimes leaked to tabloids. Also, sometimes physicians and patients made premature public appearances while the patients were still in the early stages of healing, before anyone yet knew the long-term outcome.

Mayo wanted to take a respectful approach to informing the public of any face transplant it performed. The plan was to wait until the postoperative healing was nearly complete and the outcome of the operation was better known before presenting the patient to the public—and then if, and only if, the patient wanted a public presentation.

Mardini felt grateful to the members of other surgical teams who shared their face transplant experiences in all aspects, from surgical technique to media exposure. "We learned from other teams through observations and discussions," he said. "Every transplant performed around the world is a massive undertaking and an opportunity to advance the field. We all make decisions that, at the time, seemed reasonable and appropriate. Although it's easy to observe from the outside and find faults, every team had the best interests of patients in mind. We were fortunate to gain from others' experiences and refine our procedure and process—it's what we expected to do."

On the surface, it seemed unbelievable that Mayo Clinic was considering performing its first face transplant—an enormously costly, complex, and time-consuming procedure—on a patient who had intentionally shot himself in the face during a suicide attempt. Understandably, Andy's Mayo physicians needed to ensure that their patient had moved away from any suicidal impulses and his former substance use. They worried that Andy would have trouble handling the psychological pressures of the surgery and his recovery.

Andy took advantage of Mardini's offer to introduce him to previous face transplant patients. Andy talked to one of them on the phone. "He said to do it. He said, 'Don't be afraid of anything. It's so worth it. The outcome you're going to get is unbelievable,'" Andy remembers. That reassurance helped. Based on growing evidence and the experience of others, Andy's belief that a face transplant was the right treatment for him was strengthened.

Meanwhile, Andy still had to convince the people at Mayo that he was a suitable candidate for a face transplant. That meant he had to demonstrate not only that he had the psychological and social qualities to succeed in the treatment but also that he understood the demands of a face transplant. Mardini remembers one particular visit from Andy in which he appeared to be in command of a much larger amount of information about the procedure than he had shown earlier. Andy was no longer asking them to perform the transplant on him simply because he yearned for it and trusted them. He had information that bolstered the request.

At another meeting with members of the transplant team, Andy fielded questions about the areas of facial function he hoped to gain after a transplant. "He wanted to able to kiss his nephew on the forehead, and he wanted to be able to eat potato chips," Ewoldt remembers him answering. Andy saw images of patients around the world who had undergone a face transplant and noticed the mixed outcomes. Some patients looked great and attained good facial function, and some experienced complications and disappointing outcomes. Slowly, Andy was learning enough to be able to provide informed consent.

A poor candidate for a face transplant would be a patient with facial injuries or disfigurement that could be substantially improved by conventional treatment, or someone lacking social support or emotional and intellectual maturity. Unrealistic expectations were another disqualifier. Andy was distinguishing himself from people in those groups.

In the end, Andy researched face transplant surgery and understood as much about it as any patient possibly could, reading articles, going through medical research, and talking with his physicians. The multidisciplinary VCA selection committee grew convinced that he was the right patient for the first performance of a face transplant at Mayo Clinic. He persuaded them, "which I think is remarkable given the big institution, strong reputation, and high visibility" at Mayo, Mardini says. "Our first one would be on someone who attempted suicide. Our team was able to see Andy for who he was at the time he was being considered for a face transplant, and not for who he was when he shot himself."

"Patient selection, patient selection, patient selection" was the mantra that Hatem Amer repeatedly uttered when considering candidates for face transplant. Over two and a half years, Mardini, Amer, Jowsey-Gregoire, and others met with Andy multiple times, believing they needed to get to know him as well as possible. The team wanted to ensure Andy had caregivers at home, psychiatric support, a way to manage his medicines, and sufficient inner commitment. Would he be able to adapt to the social changes and the end of isolation that his transplant would bring? How would he feel wearing a deceased donor's face? Andy even had to write an essay about why he wanted a face transplant. In the end, Andy handled the challenges and met the requirements. He was all in, as was his Mayo team.

Meanwhile, Rhonda's health had been deteriorating, to the point that she became bedridden. She had a mass the size of a fist above her heart, but it had never been biopsied. "The doctor said this thing has got to come out as soon as possible," Andy said. "And she just never did it." Often when he visited her, she slept through his time with her. Andy felt sad to see her so sick, and by 2013 he knew she had grown sick of being sick. She died on May 19, 2013, at the age of fifty-nine. He missed her support and love.

In 2014, Andy took a job with Grizzly Services in Newcastle. Yet he hadn't lost his interest in pursuing a career as an electrician. He soon landed a job as an electrician apprentice with All Electric in Gillette, Wyoming, where he worked for over a year. Eventually, as work slowed in Gillette, his company transferred him to Cheyenne, about four hours' drive from Newcastle.

# Chapter 7

# Phone Calls

———

Reconstructive plastic surgeons like Mardini often treat patients in tandem with other physicians. Their work overlaps with trauma, critical care, emergency general surgery, and other specialties. Although Mardini understood his strengths, at a place like Mayo Clinic he could also find somebody who knew more than he did about many things. Teams of surgeons and other medical providers come together to build upon one another's knowledge.

At Mayo, teams coalesce in several ways. Providers gravitate to others they like to work with. Sometimes they share an interest in the challenges of particular types of patients they treat. Or they are attracted to the way others handle themselves in their clinical work. Then, of course, certain skills are needed for specific cases. People form groups in which they can count on one another for independent thought.

Motivated by the appreciation of intellectual synergy across medical disciplines, Mardini started Mayo's facial paralysis and reanimation clinic. Its team members—surgeons, neurologists, ophthalmologists, optometrists, physical therapists, and specialists in facial nerve issues—would later play a critical role in helping Andy recover facial movement in the course that lay ahead for him.

One or two people usually lead a team. The people occupying the leadership role vary with the needs of patients. Mayo Clinic prizes people who can pull together high-quality, multidisciplinary teams that bring good results. For Andy's face transplant, Mardini and Amer assumed co-leadership of the team. Mardini was the surgical leader, and Amer took charge of medical treatment. The two physicians were vastly different types—Mardini was eager to go, while Amer was deliberate. Shirley Walter, Mardini's medical administrator, recalls once walking on the streets of Rochester with both men when they encountered a red traffic signal. "Dr. Mardini was going to cross on the red light, and Dr. Amer was standing back," she said. Those traits extended to their professional work. But the two complemented each other, and both thoughtfully and respectfully accepted the opinions of others.

Amer was well known and respected at Mayo for his thorough and methodical approach to medicine, as well as his vast knowledge of nephrology, transplant medicine, and immunosuppressive treatments. He had served medical residencies at Cairo University Hospitals and Abington Memorial Hospital in Pennsylvania, and fellowships at the Cairo Kidney Center and at Mayo Clinic College of Medicine and Science. In the years to come, Amer would be recognized by Mayo for his distinguished service as program director of the renal transplant fellowship and would become president of the International Society of Vascularized Composite Allotransplantation. He has published more than eighty papers in medical research journals.

Both Amer and Mardini wanted to learn more about the other's specialty. While Mardini and his surgical colleagues on the team set out to absorb the postoperative medical requirements for face transplant patients, Amer and his transplant physician specialists traveled and met with experts who could educate them on plastic surgery and the requirements of facial disfigurement patients.

Among those whom Mardini and Amer recruited to join the team was Elizabeth Bradley, an ophthalmologist specializing in oculoplastic surgery—one of the few ophthalmologists ever included on a face transplant team in some two dozen previous surgeries worldwide. Her main role was to protect Andy's fully functional right eye, the one that had not suffered shrapnel damage in his gunshot injury, and to ensure that the function of the eyelid and drainage of the tear glands allowed for proper eye health. "I thought it would be devastating if he had a successful face transplant but woke up blind," Bradley said. Team members like Bradley helped the others gain knowledge beyond their typical professional experience and widened their horizons. "You start appreciating more and more a patient population that you don't normally interact with," Amer said.

To others around him, Mardini's work as team co-leader seemed effortless. That was partly because his colleagues had high respect for his medical and interpersonal talents. He looked for the best in everyone he worked with. Mardini led gently, with subtlety. Many who have worked with him cannot recall an occasion when he got visibly upset or perturbed; he is bighearted and even-keeled. He diligently plans which skills he needs in fellow team members, and carefully identifies and gathers people with those skills. And hidden beneath that calm exterior is the energy he used to push through the logistics of Andy's face transplant. "It's like leading a start-up corporation," observed Mardini's team anesthesiologist, Thomas Comfere.

The multidisciplinary team Mardini and Amer had assembled for Andy's face transplant included people working in anesthesiology, nursing, social work, psychiatry, pharmacy, medical ethics, radiology, infectious diseases, dermatology, dermatopathology,

pathology, histocompatibility, physical therapy, diet and nutrition, surgery and surgical tech, photography, hospital administration, security, dentistry, and prosthetics, among other specialties. Both Amer and Mardini followed the maxim of identifying and supporting the best people for the team and then getting out of the way. They accepted criticism and suggestions. They communicated freely with each other and with the members of their team. They understood that the training of other providers was different from their own, and they valued the others for that different perspective. "He really does take advice," said team member and plastic surgeon Karim Bakri of Mardini. In turn, Mardini regarded Bakri as his chief surgical collaborator, a skilled and talented surgeon with a hunger for learning.

Another of the specialists on the team was the aforementioned prosthodontist, Thomas Salinas. Looking at Andy's case from a dental perspective, he had initially been unsure about the wisdom of performing a face transplant on Andy. Even with a donor's face that closely matched Andy's in skin coloration and bone structure, the new jaw, teeth, and other dental parts might not fit the patient well, which could cause complications and difficulties in recovery. If Andy sought a better appearance and improved function of his face, a dental mismatch might work against those goals.

Mardini understood and respected Salinas's reservations. However, if a face transplant was not undertaken, what remained of Andy's dental state could not be improved significantly. Salinas also understood that dental restoration was only a part of the benefits for Andy. The face transplant, Salinas realized, could boost Andy's entire life in terms of his relationships, social life, mental health, self-esteem, and other areas.

"It was really a phenomenal team," said certified surgical technologist Kevin Asprey, a native of southern Minnesota whose forty-year career had placed him on thousands of Mayo surgical operations. He had worked on some of Andy's reconstructive surgeries nearly ten years earlier. For the face transplant, "I never heard anyone bicker. I never heard anybody say anything negative." He was most impressed by Mardini's planning. "He had this thing planned out like I couldn't believe."

Mardini has a different interpretation of the effectiveness of the team that assembled for Andy's face transplant. To Mardini, the strongest motivation of team members was compassion and the desire to help others. Providers met Andy, "and they said, 'We want to help this guy.' Everybody was working toward helping him. They weren't taking my lead. They were pushing themselves, and we were organizing and doing it."

With a team in place, Mardini focused his attention on preparing for Andy's surgery. The weight of performing a successful face transplant on Andy was daunting, as there was no option for failure. He recalls feeling that "we had to make this as perfect as possible." Transplant nurse coordinator Lori Ewoldt had gotten the process off to an early start, beginning in 2012 to prepare a massive and complex spreadsheet, culled from initial notes and thoughts scribbled on Post-it notes, that detailed all the tasks and responsibilities needed to accomplish a face transplant. "It was a way to check and double-check," she explained. "Not that it was perfect by any means, but it was helpful."

How, for instance, do you teach a team to perform this procedure? In intense trials of surgical techniques, practice occurred over three years. On fifty Saturdays, separate from other work and responsibilities, Mardini and his surgical team worked in a cadaver lab, a place where medical staff practiced treatment techniques on donated bodies. There they built an enormously detailed map of the nerves, blood vessels, and muscle systems of the human face. While Mardini's expertise in facial nerves, facial reconstruction, and facial aesthetic surgery formed the basis of the team's knowledge of what could produce a successful face transplant, the sessions in the cadaver lab brought a deeper understanding of the under-the-skin knowledge required for the transplant team.

The group set out to understand everything they could about the workings of the face from a new perspective. The same surgeries Mardini and his partners performed every day on facial nerves to improve patients' movement and function proved helpful in anticipating the needs of Andy and other face transplant patients.

At the start, Mardini and plastic surgery partners Karim Bakri and Jorys Martinez-Jorge had entered the cadaver lab to explore and simulate variations on face transplant techniques. After many sessions they developed a unique procedure for addressing Andy's specific facial deficits. They then invited other members of the surgical team—including Uldis Bite, Basel Sharaf, and Elizabeth Bradley—to start rehearsals for the actual transplant.

Together, they studied the vital connections that allow a person to blink, grimace, smile, pucker, and chew. Using cadavers and taking videos and photos, they traced each of the nerve branches supplying every area of the face that would be transplanted. The same tracings were performed on Andy's face. At the same time, team members painstakingly planned each step of the upcoming surgery. It was going to be a medical marathon.

The cadaver lab was in the Stabile Building, a tall gray glass structure on Mayo Clinic's Rochester campus. Every Saturday, the managers of the lab would have several faces or heads ready for the team to work on. Initially, four to six team members would gather in the lab in the early morning, often staying well into the afternoon. Later the group swelled to twenty to thirty participants. The place was lively, full of discussion. Team members often referred to photos of Andy's face and a mockup of his facial defects. Depending on the focus of the day's session, the group would set up a staged facsimile of one aspect of the transplant surgery using the cadavers.

During the early sessions, team members delved deep into anatomy books, focusing on specific steps that might be necessary to take during the procurement of the donor's face and Andy's transplant. Later sessions used surgical hardware and imaging to test specific techniques and procedures. Using markers, they drew trial locations of incisions on the cadavers and tried different cuts. In one extended discussion, for instance, the cadaver lab investigators debated potential challenges in procuring the donor's jaw. Although brain dead, the donor would still have a beating heart and need to be supported by an artificial ventilator. The placement of the intubation tube connecting the donor to the ventilator would make it difficult to access critical structures in the donor's face. It would also be challenging for anaplastologists to create a prosthesis to cover the donor's face after procurement. "There were all these practical aspects that we had to think through," remembered Elizabeth Bradley. Sessions were recorded on video so that the participants could review them later.

Bradley, with a subspecialty in plastic and reconstructive surgery of the eye socket and eyelids, spent intensive time in the lab on the anatomy of tear drainage. She had found nothing in the medical literature about any previous efforts during a face transplant to reconstruct the tear drainage system from the eyes to the nose. In addition, Mardini and Bradley devoted lab time to studying how best to reconstruct the floor of Andy's eye sockets, using uninjured cheekbones from Andy's face that would be moved and reshaped to create and contour orbital bones that would take the exact shape of his original orbital floor—the thin bones that provide support for the eyes.

Training with actual human faces from cadavers was essential. According to Mardini, without these generous donations, his team would not have been as well prepared for the surgery as they ultimately were. After working fifty Saturdays in the cadaver lab studying more than forty faces and heads, team members built up the critical experience needed to execute a face transplant for the first time. The surgical team could manipulate tissues in the cadaver lab with the knowledge that their mistakes would cause no harm, all the while gaining experience that was impossible to replicate otherwise. Each minute spent in the cadaver lab offered a chance to improve.

The intense hours in the cadaver lab also revealed the value and dedication of each member of the surgical team. Some Saturdays, surgical technologists, nurse anesthetists, anesthesiologists, and operating room nurses joined the group to observe and practice, as well as take part in the workflow and experience the vibe of the team.

Mardini remembers feeling unprepared in the earliest of the cadaver lab sessions. Despite team members' knowledge of anatomy, "we knew so little about what we should do and how we should start," he said. They researched medical journal articles and "just started doing stuff."

In one example, Mardini's team investigated the course of the internal maxillary artery (IMA), a blood vessel that originates from the external carotid artery and runs below the cheekbones along each side of the face. It provides blood laterally to the maxillary bones and is a major source of blood supply to the bones of the upper jaw. It branches to smaller vessels less than one millimeter in width. Mardini and his team wanted to understand the course of that vessel and its exact anatomy and branching patterns. Could the IMA be included in the tissue dissected from the face transplant donor? This vessel was but one of countless blood channels and nerve pathways that the team had to explore, learn, and master in connecting.

For Marissa Suchyta, a research fellow working with Mardini's team, the sessions in the cadaver lab were a memorable part of her early medical career. Entering the lab for the first time, she saw two cadaver heads mounted for study. The setup of the lab struck her as professional, clean, and efficient. It was like walking into a brightly lit and well-equipped operating room. A pair of piezoelectric saws, high-tech tools for cutting bone, drew her attention, along with other equipment. The intensity of the investigations into facial anatomy, as well as the strong motivations of team members who were giving up their weekends and time with family, impressed her. The donation of time also impressed Mardini, who choked up with emotion when he remembered all the people who sacrificed personal time to a project that could have suddenly disappeared if Andy had changed his mind or suffered a medical setback before transplant.

Suchyta felt excited to be included, and the experience whetted her interest in plastic surgery as a specialty. "I really learned a lot about anatomy of the face very quickly," she said. "I learned facial nerves, bone structure on the fly those first few months." For the first time she realized the huge undertaking of a face transplant. "Seeing a cadaver's face essentially come off made me think initially, 'Oh my gosh, this is crazy in a lot of ways.'" During her second week in the lab, she met Andy and better understood the challenges of his life and the difficulties he was having with a reconstructed face, along with his commitment to undergoing a face transplant. "That made me understand what a huge impact this would have on someone's life and why someone would want to go through this extensive surgery and recovery."

A critical activity in the cadaver lab over those many weekends was the team members' growing expertise with tools called cutting guides. The guides fit over the faces of both patient and donor and had slits that helped the surgeons make their cuts with precision. Andy's cutting guides were customized to the exact dimensions of his face. But the surgical cuts on the yet unknown donor would depend on the size of the head and dimensions of the face.

Another useful tool the team had access to was three-dimensional imaging and modeling. Mardini was familiar with this technology, having used it to prepare for head and neck re-constructive surgeries for many years and pioneering its use in surgeries to reshape children's cranial bones. Using information from CT scans, including an old CT scan of Andy's face taken prior to his injury, the transplant team used 3D modeling to create and print three-dimensional models of Andy's future face. This was a big help in planning for the transplant. In addition, Mardini and his team tapped 3D Corporation, a company that had assisted Mardini before, to develop face transplant protocols and guides with great precision.

The gains made in the cadaver lab were often slow and incre-mental. The cutting guides needed modifications, sometimes major ones. The teams made decisions about which tools to use in the actual transplant—choosing between the piezoelectric saws and more traditional bone saws, for example, for specific stages of the work.

Just as important as the anatomical and surgical problems discussed in the cadaver lab were the human bonds formed there among team members. "If you're sitting there with somebody working on a skull for two hours and you talk to them about their kids and their vacation, what else they're working on, and all that, you get to know them as people," Bradley said. Over lunch, they all shared stories.

Time together in the cadaver lab forged an especially close connection between Mardini and Bakri. The latter was younger and had been a member of Mayo's faculty for three years compared with Mardini's ten; he too had grown up in Beirut, Lebanon, in a close-knit culture of family connections, generosity, and hospitality that led him to often think about the needs of others as a first impulse. It was remarkably like Mardini's formative childhood environment. Bakri calls their bond "a grassroots sort of friendship, almost like kids who grow up together at school." Sometimes after a lab session was over, Mardini would leave the building, join Bakri in his car, and drive around for an hour or two. They would drive into the countryside outside Rochester and then back into the city. At other times they just parked and talked in the car. They reviewed what had happened that day in the lab and what they should try next time. In addition to keeping detailed notebooks covering all that took place in the lab, they fixed in their minds what they had learned through their discussions with each other. They bounced ideas back and forth. They debated new approaches to overcoming anatomical problems and picked which to try in the lab. "I think that was really, really a good thing," Bakri said.

Through his attention to building strong teamwork in the cadaver lab and ensuring everyone on the team understood the planning for the transplant, Mardini encouraged the team to think beyond their customary roles. He asked team members, for instance, to consider how to tag Andy's facial nerve branches so that they could be properly identified and connected to the face donor's corresponding nerves.

Meanwhile, Lori Schacht, the nurse manager in the operating room with responsibility for assigning nurses and surgical technologists and making sure surgical preparations went smoothly on the day of the transplant, gathered all the supplies and instrumentation needed to perform the face transplant. Participating in team discussions led by Mardini gave Schacht a good idea of what was ahead. "I had to think outside the box a lot because we'd never done anything like that," she said. "For instance, how would we keep all of the individual facial nerves identified during the operation? How were we going to protect Andy [from bedsores] during this lengthy procedure by moving his extremities during the surgery?" In addition, Schacht would have to staff two operating rooms: one for Andy and one for the donor.

Schacht, who grew up in nearby Pine Island, Minnesota, had spent eighteen years as a surgical technologist in the operating rooms at Mayo and was well prepared for these responsibilities.

She once worked on a team that reconstructed a patient whose face had been sheared off in a car accident.

~

During these preparations, Andy was being readied for his central role in the transplant surgery. His overall health was evaluated several times. Mayo physicians noted that his gunshot injury had left him with a diminished sense of smell, poor vision in his left eye, difficulty chewing and swallowing, and trouble enunciating the letters *P* and *S*. Occasionally he felt the ghostly sensation of the tip of his missing nose itching. He had symptoms of depression, including a tendency to be hard on himself. He had stopped drinking, smoking, and using marijuana. Even so, Mayo wanted him to go through four weeks of outpatient chemical dependency treatment, and he completed it successfully in 2014. He told psychiatrist Sheila Jowsey-Gregoire, whom he was working with, that his abstinence was "the best thing I have done."

By the same token, Amer, Mardini, and the VCA team's social workers worked hard to continue to educate Andy on the risks of face transplant, the necessity and potential complications of immunosuppression, and the lifestyle changes—such as avoiding excessive sun, soil, and dust—he would have to follow. And Andy's transplant team repeated the dangers of the failure of the transplant, a rejection of the graft, which could leave him much worse off than he was now. They considered him well informed regarding all possible complications. Andy asked if, after the transplant, he would be able to use a motocross bike to ride trails with his friends. Due to a possible weakening of his bones from immunosuppression medication and the hazards of dirt and dust, Amer advised against it.

Since 2015, Andy had been working as an electrician, and he enjoyed hunting, fishing, snowmobiling, cribbage, and working on his truck. He avoided situations that might lead to drinking alcohol and smoking marijuana. He regularly saw a therapist. Although Andy lived alone, he made efforts to get out and spend time with friends. Unexpectedly, he told his Mayo social worker that he enjoyed his life now more than before he shot himself. He felt, he told her, "deeply grateful to be alive." After the transplant, Andy said, he would be willing to take up to a year off from work during his recovery. Such a hiatus might be financially difficult, however.

Though Rhonda and Andy's father, Reed, now retired, had split up some years earlier, Reed reappeared as a supportive figure in Andy's life. The worst thing Andy could imagine after his face transplant was waking up alone, without anyone to take an interest in him. But Reed was eager to serve as Andy's family caregiver after the transplant. "This is what he wants," Reed said. "And I want what he wants." He added: "I ain't stressed about it one bit." Reed was planning on staying for months in Rochester to help with his son's recovery. Andy realized he would need some time separate from his father after the surgery, but he thought his father's interest was "pretty cool," as he told a social worker, and he welcomed Reed's involvement. His dad's diabetes and other health problems might prevent him from doing all he wanted to, in which case Andy hoped to rely on a combination of his siblings and friends for help and support. These would include the owners of the lodge where Andy had previously worked, Larry and Twylla.

To be properly matched to a donor, Andy needed to be screened for several common viruses. One was cytomegalovirus (CMV), a virus normally inconsequential in people other than those who are pregnant or have immunological weaknesses. Because Andy would be immunologically suppressed after his transplant, it was important that his donor matched him in exposure to CMV. Another infectious agent, Epstein-Barr virus (EBV), the frequent cause of mononucleosis in people, posed graver risks. In an immunosuppressed state, catching EBV from a donor's tissues could have serious consequences, possibly sparking the growth of malignant cancers in Andy's lymphatic system. Andy had long thought he'd come down with mononucleosis as a teenager, but no physician had ever diagnosed it in him.

As it happened, in screening, Andy tested negative for both CMV and EBV, an unusual combination. This meant Andy had never been exposed to either virus, despite his recollection of having had mononucleosis. These results placed him in a distinct minority of Americans, of whom 50 to 80 percent have had exposure to CMV and three-quarters have had exposure to EBV. It was clear to Andy's transplant team that finding a donor who likewise tested negative for both CMV and EBV would be ideal, but holding out for such a match likely meant a waiting time that would be too long.

Mayo's infectious disease expert on the transplant team, Raymund Razonable, advised that while a mismatch on EBV would raise unacceptable risks, such as blood cancer, a CMV mismatch might be manageable. Amer believed that Andy should wait until an EBV-negative donor became available. Statistically, three-quarters of possible donors were suddenly out of reach.

LifeSource, Mayo's organ procurement partner in the Upper Midwest, pulled statistics that helped Andy's team determine the likely wait time for a donor: two years. Once a donor candidate appeared, Andy's fate would hang on the decision of the donor's family. Would a donation of facial tissues accord with the family's cultural and religious beliefs? Would it make them uncomfortable? Everyone at Mayo hoped a donor would emerge whose family agreed with a sentiment common among people working in transplants: "Don't take your organs to heaven. God knows we need them here on Earth."

Unwilling to have so many potential donors unavailable to him because of his EBV-negative status, Andy tried an unsanctioned method of exposing himself to EBV in advance of his transplant.

"I found somebody who had mono and had them drink out of a soda can," he said. Then he drank from the same can. It did not work; he remained healthy and unexposed to the virus that is so common in our society. Amer did not approve of this attempted self-infection: "Willingly trying to infect himself carries the risk of untoward viruses, and I cannot recommend such a practice due to those concerns," he wrote in the medical record.

Andy was being mentally prepared for a face transplant as well. Jowsey-Gregoire and others working in psychiatry at Mayo continued to work with him in terms of his psychological stability, history of chemical dependence, family support, understanding of the transplant process, and ability to emerge successfully from the extensive rehabilitation that would be needed. When Andy told his transplant team that he feared "being sick all the time" from immunosuppressive medications, they worked to help him reduce his apprehension. They wanted him to be able to problem-solve when faced with the inevitable challenges ahead and learn how to be flexible and optimistic. Jowsey-Gregoire aimed to support Andy in reintegrating into his life fully and without guilt over his past struggles and without a feeling of indebtedness for the opportunity of a face transplant.

By December 2014, Andy's placement on the official face transplant waiting list seemed close at hand. "He has very realistic expectations and understands his CMV negative and EBV negative status may prolong his waiting time," a social worker noted in his medical record. "I am ready," Andy told Jowsey-Gregoire. "I know I am ready."

Even so, well into 2015 Amer and Mardini were continuing to assess Andy's suitability as a face transplant recipient. They conferred with Mayo's VCA selection committee to come to a final decision. At last it came: "The team feels comfortable that the patient is an appropriate candidate for a face transplantation both from a medical-surgical as well as a psychologic standpoint," Mardini wrote on April 3. "Patient has the appropriate support network to proceed with this type of procedure."

Three days later, Andy signed a form giving his informed consent to the transplant surgery. On a visit to Mayo several weeks later, he spoke of his contentment with his decision to proceed. It was the first time he had come to Rochester without feeling nervous. "I was excited to come. I feel so comfortable with all of you," Andy told social worker Clare Dudzinski.

Just in case, Mardini devised a contingency plan to fall back on if the transplant failed. He and his team would use tissue transfers from the thigh, bone flaps from the fibula, and other grafts to repair the massive damage to Andy's face that was possible if all went wrong with the transplant.

In the summer of 2015, Andy's official listing in the transplant waiting pool had not yet cleared all its hurdles. "Our plan is to list the patient soon," Mardini wrote in the record, though by the middle of January 2016 that had not yet occurred. With the listing undoubtedly coming soon, Mayo's social workers wanted to ensure that Andy could move quickly when notification came that a donor was available.

At this time Andy was living in Cheyenne, Wyoming, in an apartment near his employer, and he spent some weekends in his trailer home in Newcastle. He assured the social workers that he would accept no job assignments that would take him far from home and would forgo all hunting and fishing trips that would make it difficult to contact him. Mayo let him know they would charter a plane to pick him up in either Cheyenne or Newcastle when a donor appeared. However, no one had yet worked out the seemingly minor detail of how Andy would travel from the Rochester airport to Saint Marys. Andy volunteered to take a taxicab, but the social workers believed doing so would endanger the discreet approach that Mayo had planned for Andy's surgery. Eventually, everyone agreed that Andy would travel from the airport to the hospital by ambulance.

Andy's transplant team had the luxury of benefiting from the face transplant experiences of teams at other institutions. While Mayo's team members respected the pioneering efforts of their colleagues around the world, they saw the many unexpected results of patients whose privacy had been compromised too early or too much. The early release of photos could distract from Andy's recovery and could even cause him humiliation. With Andy's agreement, the Mayo team would try to control Andy's story as much as possible to preserve his dignity and confidentiality. In the spirit of sharing scientific information that would benefit others, the medical and scientific communities could publish photos and stories in peer-reviewed journals. But to allow the public distribution of graphic photos in the midst of Andy's preparation for face transplant and recovery was not a path Mayo wanted to follow.

At last, on January 25, 2016, Andy's name landed on the VCA transplant waiting list. "By the time we listed him, everybody on the team felt like this is the right guy [for a transplant], and Andy felt like he was doing the right thing," said Brooks Edwards, director of Mayo Clinic's Transplant Center, who was born in Rochester and spent decades at Mayo as a specialist in heart transplantation. "He was all in, and the team was all in." Andy told his relatives and close friends about his anticipation of a face transplant, and he made sure they also knew about his expectations of privacy: there would be no social media sharing regarding his forthcoming surgery. He and Mayo intended to keep the face transplant quiet, whenever it happened, until they mutually decided to make it public.

Quickly, LifeSource, a regional center for organ, tissue, and eye donation, sprang into action. Headquartered in Minneapolis, LifeSource managed all donations throughout its area of coverage— Minnesota, North Dakota, South Dakota, and western Wisconsin— including transporting donors to organ procurement sites. (In such a geographically large region, LifeSource often chartered airplanes for rapid delivery of its precious cargo.) It also provided education on organ donations and gave support to donor families.

Typically, LifeSource's direct involvement in an organ procurement in its region—except in the case of kidneys and other tissues that can be procured from a living donor—begins when a physician declares an organ donor brain dead according to established neurological criteria. Then the agency and its organ preservationists take over, with one donor often being the source of several organ procurements. LifeSource continues to give support to the family of the donor, sometimes for decades.

Meg Rogers, then director of transplant center relations for LifeSource, had worked for the organization for decades. Earlier, as an ICU nurse at Hennepin County Medical Center in Minneapolis, she once cared for a patient who became an organ donor, an experience that moved and fascinated her. After providing care for a second patient who became a donor, Rogers saw an ad for a job at LifeSource. It was a different organization then: only a few dozen employees, a lot of paperwork, little technology, and busy telephones. She began as a donation coordinator, helping donor families in the intensive care unit when a donor was declared brain dead. She advanced to become director of procurement and led all LifeSource's organ operations and teams. Eventually the staff quadrupled in size and the organization built a larger headquarters as the demand for organs increased. In her role as director, Rogers worked to build its relationships with the region's nine transplant centers.

Mayo's creation of its face transplant program and its listing of Andy as a waiting face transplant recipient were the first such notifications LifeSource had ever received. Ewoldt had earlier called Rogers to broach the subject. Mayo was going to work on a face transplant program, she told Rogers. "There was a very pregnant pause, and she said, 'What face transplant program?'" Ewoldt recalled. "We occasionally have a chuckle over that."

Despite her reaction, Rogers was not surprised to see this development. "Mayo is a very patient-driven organization, and you see that in everything they do," she said. Their existing transplant programs were strong, and the institution knew how to make an additional program happen. Yet VCA-derived transplants were relatively new, and willing donors did not tend to think in advance of donating hands or faces. LifeSource had yet to approach a donor or family about making a VCA donation.

Andy needed a male donor with similar skin tone, a compatible blood type, and a matching EBV-negative status; furthermore, the donor could be no more than ten years older than Andy, who was thirty in 2016. Mardini worried the wait could last years. Finding the right donor was like locating a particular blade of grass on a plush lawn. In addition to these restrictive parameters, any potential donation had to come from someone who had been declared brain dead but whose heart was still beating. Brain death means the donor's brain functions, including those of the brain stem, have ceased. Respiration, blood circulation, and other essential functions can be mechanically maintained. (Legally, brain death is the same as cardiac death.)

"People have an image of a motorcycle accident, and someone's dead at the scene, and now you're going to get their kidneys," Brooks Edwards said. That scenario plays out "only in the movies." A donor involved in an accident or other health mishap must be resuscitated and taken to a hospital. In the ICU, they are placed on a ventilator. After many medical interventions, a neurologist ultimately finds the donor has lost all brain function, and the donor is declared brain dead. "When that happens, it triggers a mandatory request for organ donation to the family," Edwards said, even when the patient has previously indicated a willingness to donate organs, on a driver's license or elsewhere. Because face and hand donations are relatively new, it cannot be assumed that everyone who agreed to be an organ donor knew about these types of donations. Approval to procure hands or a face must come from the donor's family.

When a donor emerges, the organ transplant system checks the patient waiting list. Patients receive priority based on the severity of their illness and their need for a specific organ. There will always be matches, often many, for livers, kidneys, and lungs. Organs may be offered to twenty different hospital transplant programs, and the top-ranked patients on the waiting list will get them. In nearly all regions of the United States, however, few patients are on the waiting list for faces. Often there's only one patient waiting, or none. Andy was the only patient awaiting a face in his region.

In the spring of 2016, news was coming out about a face transplant patient on the East Coast who was experiencing tissue rejection. Jowsey-Gregoire told Andy to contact Amer if this news sparked any worries about the transplant he was anticipating receiving. Andy felt confident, however. He knew that every step in the surgery had been thought out a thousand times. Everyone—Andy's medical caregivers, family, and close friends—understood the goals of the face transplant, and all were determined to accompany him to the finish line, and past it. They had seen him struggle and persevere despite the difficulties of his life. His goals were to have a functional face and to be able to walk into a room and talk to people without a new acquaintance asking him what was wrong with his face.

The details were falling into place. Andy's social workers asked him how he wanted to pass his time in the hospital while recovering from his surgery. He speculated that he could watch movies on his laptop computer, talk on the phone with friends, and use the internet. Pressed about what intellectually engaging activities he might prefer, he offered to work on his hobby of building model airplanes, among other pursuits.

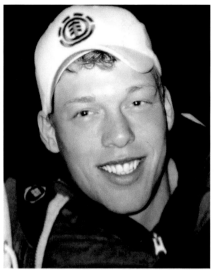

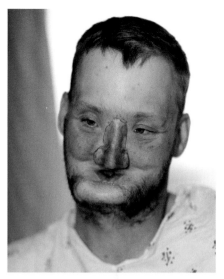

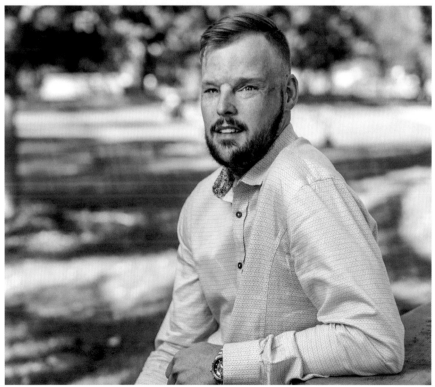

The three faces Andy has had in his lifetime. Top left, clockwise: Andy before injury; Andy after injury, immediately before his face transplant in 2016; Andy after the procedure in 2020.

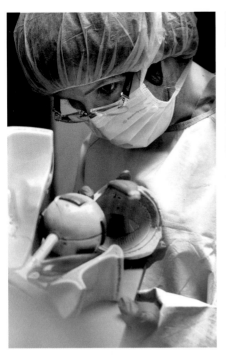

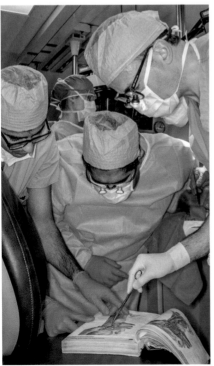

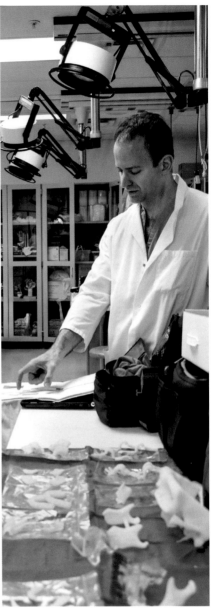

Before the face transplant, Samir Mardini (right) and his medical team researched and rehearsed the procedure for approximately three years, including over 50 Saturdays.

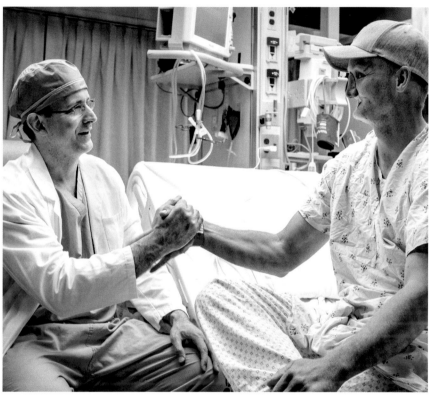

Mardini and Andy connect the night before the transplant surgery, following the discussion of the risks of the procedure. The surgery took place June 11-13, 2016.

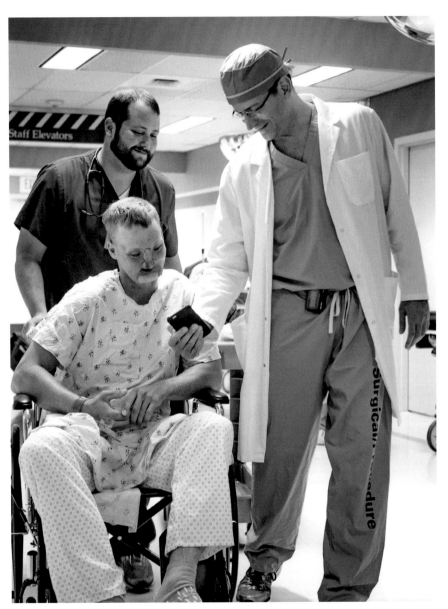

Keeping the mood light, Mardini shares videos of his children with Andy as they make their way to the operating room.

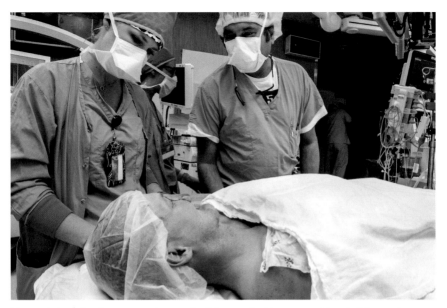

Years later, Andy remembers climbing onto the operating table and beseeching the nurse, "Please don't let anything bad happen to me."

"Don't you worry about that," she replied.

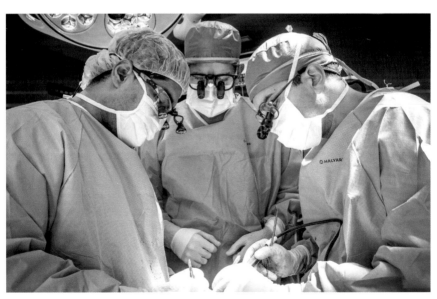

Jorys Martinez-Jorge (left) and Karim Bakri (right) assist Mardini (center) in the first phase of the transplant, which involved removing the face of Andy's donor, Calen "Rudy" Ross.

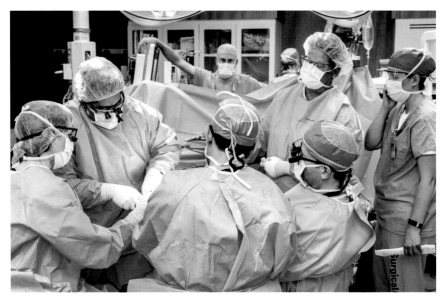

The multiday procedure required a highly complex level of teamwork.

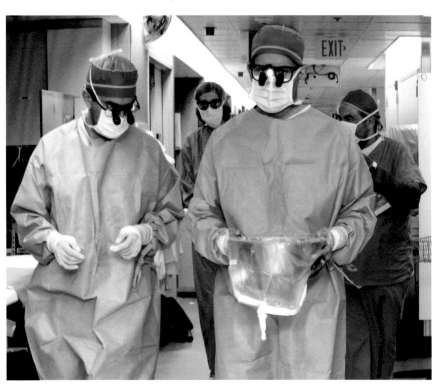

Transporting the donor tissue to Andy's suite.

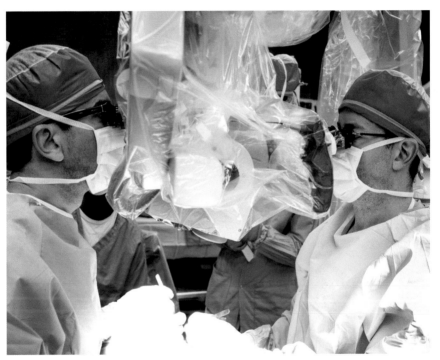

Bakri (left) and Mardini (right) use powerful microscopes to help them connect fine nerves and blood vessels.

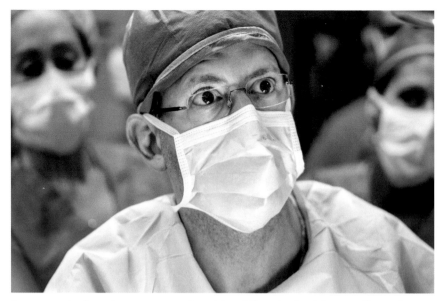

A moment of panic emerges when blood flow to Andy's new face stops and the skin drastically turns white. The team discovers a blood vessel spasm deep within the tissue.

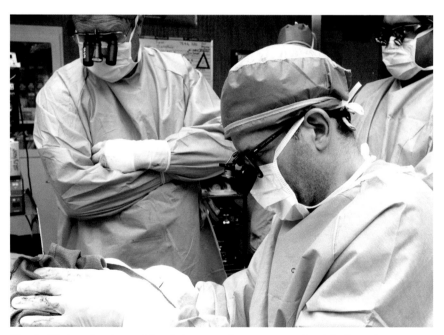

Final stitches in place, Mardini manually squeezes Andy's face to reduce postsurgical inflammation.

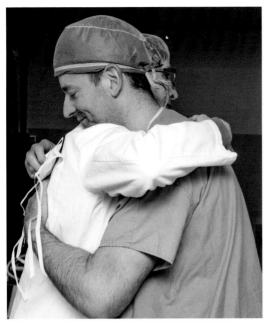

On completion of the transplant, more than 50 hours after it began, a stubbled but joyful Mardini embraces fellow surgeon Elizabeth Bradley.

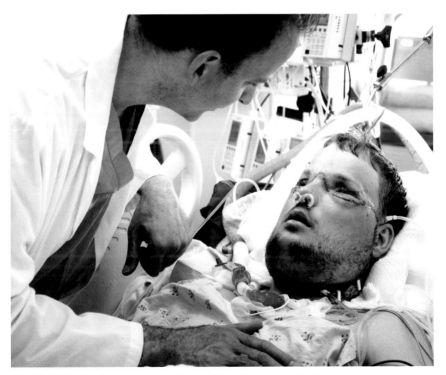

Mardini greets Andy several days after the transplant surgery.

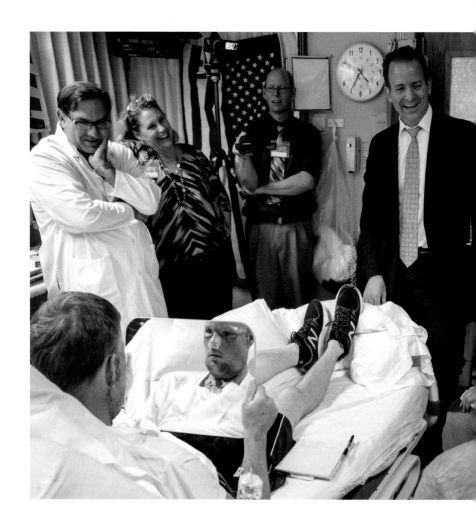

Andy, accompanied by his brother, Ronald,
father, Reed, and Mayo staff, looks at his
new face for the first time in a mirror. Still
unable to speak or make facial expressions,
he describes his reaction in writing.

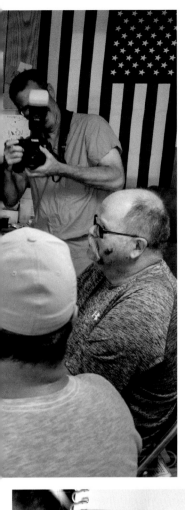

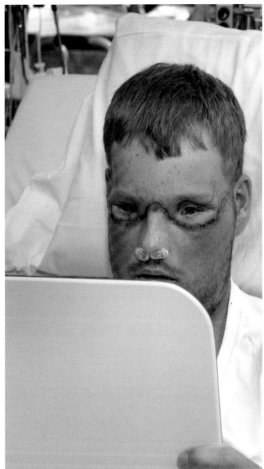

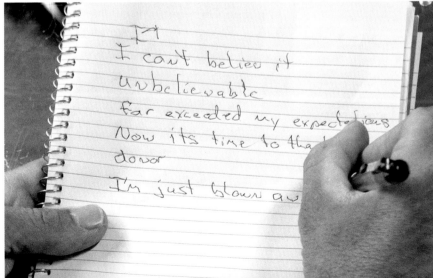

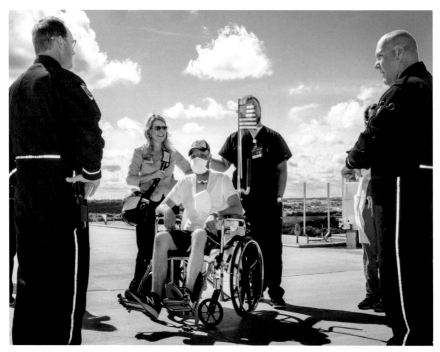

While in recovery, Andy takes a field trip to see Mayo's helicopter pad.

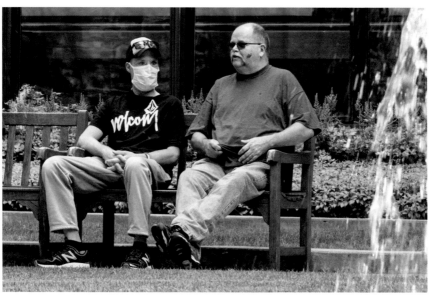

Andy enjoys some fresh air on Mayo's campus with his father, Reed, who stayed in Rochester with Andy for several months.

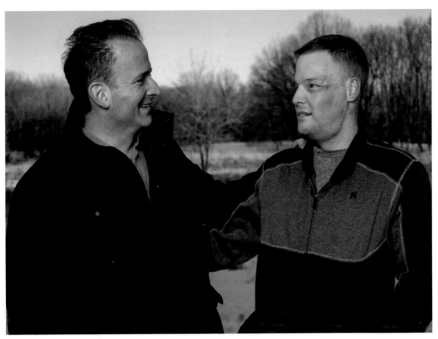

Mardini and Andy less than a year after the transplant.

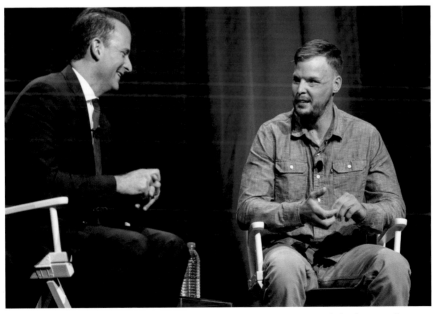

Mardini and Andy appear together onstage, sharing Andy's dramatic story of transformation, in 2019.

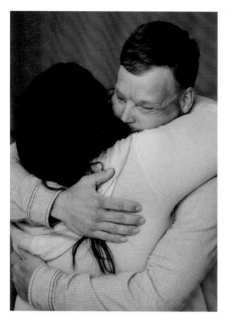
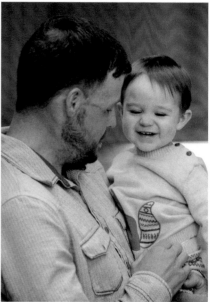
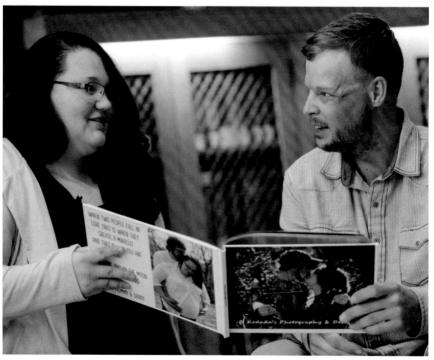

Andy meets Lilly Ross (now Lilly Warborg), Rudy's wife, and Lilly and Rudy's young son in 2017.

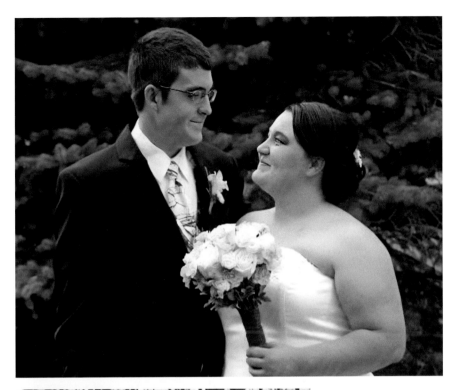

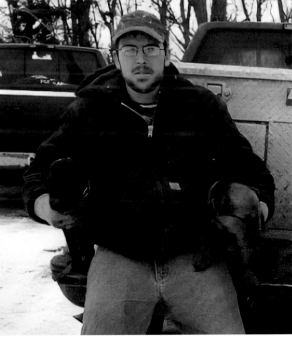

Some of Lilly's favorite photos of Rudy — on their wedding day and with his dogs.

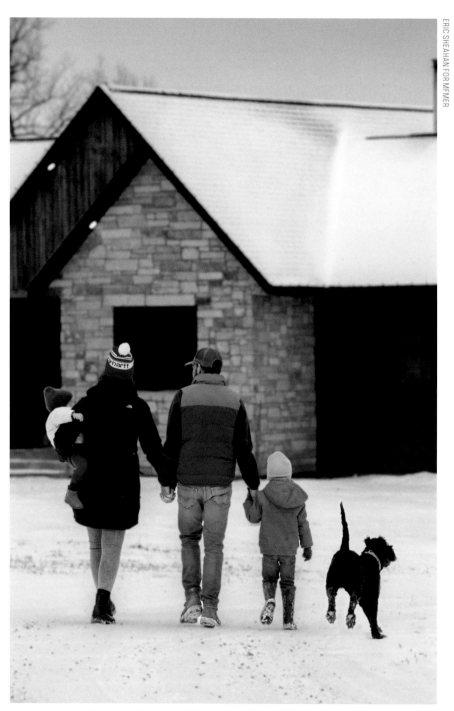

Kim, Andy, and their children in 2025, in front of the home they built together.

~

A few months after Andy was listed, on Tuesday, June 7, 2016, Hatem Amer received a phone call. A possible donor had entered the system. "My assumption was that it was going to be one of many phone calls to come," Amer said, because all donors required extensive screening. "We had calculated that there would [likely] be only two donors suitable for Andy over twenty-four months. You wouldn't expect that the first phone call you get, they'd say, 'We think we might have a suitable donor.'" The donor, who had died by suicide, had suffered no structural damage to the face that would limit the availability of tissues Andy needed for his transplant. Amer noted that not all the match testing had been completed, and so he asked for the tissue type and other test results.

Mardini also received a notification from LifeSource. Was Mayo interested in pursuing the possibility? "The answer was yes, for sure," Mardini remembered, "but I thought this donor would not be the one because it was the first call we had gotten." What were the odds that the first offer would prove acceptable?

When the match testing checked out, the next step was to gain approval from the donor's family to use their loved one's face for a transplant. Because they had never before posed the question, nobody at LifeSource knew how a donor's family would react to this request.

What was the most sensitive way to ask a family for a face donation? How to raise the subject and continue the conversation? LifeSource's staff consulted colleagues in the New England area, where a couple of face transplants had recently occurred. "What we learned, and what we always knew, was that families are resilient and want to share a legacy," Meg Rogers of LifeSource said. "If the donor meets the qualifications, we should talk with that family and give them the opportunity." If the family felt uncertain that the donor would have approved of bequeathing their face, or if they worried that the transplanted face might be recognizable (an unlikely possibility), they could say no. Otherwise, they could agree to make a donation.

The conversation between LifeSource and the donor's family about a face donation occurred on June 8, and after a few hours of deliberation the family decided to give the gift of a face. A CT scan of the face was made and sent to Mardini's team, which could use it to begin its planning and perform three-dimensional modeling. Conventional photos of the donor's face sent chills down Mardini's spine. "He was the perfect match by skin color, structure, shape, and age," Mardini said. "If they were to walk into a store together, you would think they were cousins."

The situation looked perfect until tests showed that the donor was CMV-positive, unlike Andy. This was not ideal, Mardini thought, but the team's infectious disease expert, Raymund Razonable, had already determined that a CMV mismatch would be manageable and that the risk of the donor's strain of CMV being resistant to antiviral medications was low. The plastic surgeon was about to embark on travel to Las Vegas, a work trip plus vacation time with his wife and two children. "We needed to make a decision about our trip, so after discussion with the surgical team we decided to head to the airport. If necessary, we could head back home if the donor situation required it," Mardini said.

On the way to the Twin Cities airport, seventy-five miles from Rochester, Mardini held conference calls and discussions with Amer, Edwards, and Razonable. Running late at the airport, Mardini hurriedly checked their bags. He and his family passed through the security checkpoint even as a conference call was ongoing. To the Mardini children's delight, a man appeared with a golf cart to rush them to their gate. The group arrived with only two minutes to spare before the plane's doors would close. Mardini was still on the phone waiting for a final decision from the team. His wife, Rawan, could see a succession of emotions appear on his face. The gate agent agreed to hold off on closing the door for an additional thirty seconds.

After a thorough examination of the donor's medical history and discussion of potential implications, Razonable gave his recommendation to proceed with the donation and transplant. Amer, Edwards, and Mardini all agreed. The transplant was on—and the trip to Las Vegas was off. Within minutes, Mardini and his family were back in their car, although their luggage was already on its way to Vegas. Mardini was headed back to Rochester, ready to undertake an entirely new professional challenge.

That same Wednesday, June 8, at 6:00 p.m., more than eight hundred miles from Mayo Clinic, Andy received a phone call from Mardini while he was filling a tire on his car after changing a flat. "What are you doing?" Mardini asked. Andy told Mardini he was filling his tire. "Good," Mardini replied. Andy was initially puzzled—how could having a flat tire be good? Then Andy's thoughts took a turn. He felt chills and the hair stood up on his arms as he realized this must be it. Just then Mardini said there might be a suitable donor available now. Stunned, Andy wanted to know something about the donor and his family, but Mardini could give no details. He instructed Andy to prepare to leave for Rochester soon.

Andy finished working on the tire and made calls to his father, his brother, and his friend Larry, along with a few others. In his little apartment, he did laundry and packed for his trip. He called his workplace, where a couple of coworkers knew he was listed for a face transplant, to tell them he might be away for a while. At this point, Andy felt ready to begin the next stage of his life. He was also prepared for the possibility that it might not happen—for the donor's family to decline, for example, or for something else to fall through. "If not, then I got a ton of clean clothes," he said. He heard nothing more from Mardini that night. Thinking the right donor would come along when it was supposed to happen, he went to work the next morning. He said prayers for the donor's family and for himself. He knew someone had to die for a donor's face to become available, and he felt bad about wanting that.

Andy was on the job digging a ditch with an excavator when he received a call from a Mayo social worker. She gave the news that the donor's spouse had approved donating the face for Andy's transplant, along with many other organs that would go to additional recipients. "You've got to get on a plane right now," she told him. "I can't," he protested. "I have a ditch opened up." Then he thought for a moment, and said, "I have to backfill it real quick. Then I'll get on the plane."

He filled the ditch and went home. After calling the people closest to him to tell them that a donor's face was waiting for him, he went to the airport and waited for his plane to arrive. He watched some hockey on the TV in the waiting area and then ran into a friend he knew casually from the gym. The man asked where he was going. "I can't tell you," Andy said. "But I can tell you that you won't recognize me when I get back." Puzzled, his friend asked, "What does that mean?" Andy repeated that he could not tell him.

Meanwhile, in voicemail messages that some recipients saved for years, members of the face transplant team heard from transplant nurse coordinator Lori Ewoldt that a donor and Andy himself were on their way to Rochester. Ewoldt and other members of the team placed some of the calls and sent some texts late at night, requesting transplant team members to report for work on Friday, June 10, or in the early hours of Saturday, June 11.

In Wyoming, waiting for his plane to take off, Andy had a difficult phone conversation with his brother, Ronald. Andy knew it would be a long surgery and there were risks. Although it is uncommon, people die having knee surgery, hip surgery—any kind of surgery. He had no idea what was going to happen. "If something does happen to me," he told Ronald, "I want you to take everything—it's yours for the taking." Andy teared up but tried not to cry. He said he could not talk about it more and ended the call.

In Sioux Falls, South Dakota, the donor was also beginning a trip to Rochester. Calen "Rudy" Ross was an outgoing and adventurous outdoorsman from the town of Fulda, Minnesota, who loved hunting and fishing. Struggling with depression, he shot himself at the age of twenty-one, the same age at which Andy had attempted suicide. Andy had shot himself with a shotgun positioned below the jaw; he destroyed his face but did not die. Rudy had placed the gun to his left temple. He died but did not injure his face except for a small bruise that developed in his left lower eyelid from the impact of the bullet. He left behind his new wife, nineteen-year-old Lilly Ross, who was eight months pregnant. They had been high school sweethearts. Earlier, Rudy had indicated on his driver's license that his heart, liver, kidneys, and lungs would be available for donation.

A LifeSource representative had asked Lilly if she was willing to help a young man who was on the waiting list for a face transplant. She was initially skeptical, afraid of someday seeing her husband's face on another man. Assured, however, that the transplant would involve removing bone and tissue below Rudy's eyes and that nobody would recognize his face, she spoke to a close friend of Rudy's, who thought Rudy would have approved of the donation. Despite her grief at her husband's death, Lilly quickly gave permission. More than anything, she hoped that her unborn child would someday appreciate how his dad had helped so many people. (Lilly remarried in 2024 and is now Lilly Warborg.)

Andy's two-and-a-half-hour flight to Rochester gave him time to think about what was coming—or to avoid thinking about it. He gazed out at the afternoon sky and tried to stop ruminating about the surgery. "I remember flying over the Twin Cities, looking out over them, just enjoying life the last little bit because this could have been my last trip—who knew?" he said. He tried to take his mind off the possibility of something bad happening during the surgery. He trusted Mardini completely, yet it was difficult to keep doubts from filtering through his mind.

To preserve Andy's privacy, the ambulance staff who would be picking him up at the airport did not know about his impending face transplant. However, when the ambulance arrived, Andy was nowhere to be found. Lynette Fix, a transplant nurse coordinator who was aboard the ambulance with Lori Ewoldt, placed a call to his cellphone and learned that his flight had arrived early. Seeing no one there to pick him up, Andy had hopped into a taxi. Fix asked him where the taxi was. Looking out the cab window, Andy said he could see a sign for a Kohl's store in the distance. Fix knew exactly where that store was. She told Andy to head for the Kohl's parking lot, where everyone would rendezvous.

Around 11:00 p.m. Andy met up with the members of his transplant team in the parking lot. "Andy jumps out, we hug him, and we all jump into the ambulance," Ewoldt remembered. "We sit there and stare at one another for a moment, and then we all just burst out laughing." Andy said, "You guys almost lost me." Ewoldt replied: "Andy, can we just never speak of this again?" His relieved reply was, "Yeah, not a chance."

The prelude to Andy's face transplant had begun.

# Chapter 8

# Adjoining Suites

———

A ndy felt calm when he checked into the Rochester hotel where he would spend the night before his face transplant began. He no longer felt scared. Focused on the surgery, he forgot to check on the outcome of the NHL Stanley Cup championship game that day, diehard sports fan though he was. As he prepared for bed, he strove to relax and mentally prepare himself for the momentous event ahead.

The next morning, Ewoldt walked Andy the short distance from the hotel to Saint Marys. She was relieved to have been able to share some laughs with him the previous night after the ambulance finally made its rendezvous with his taxicab. It was hard not to look at him through a mother's eyes. He was young enough to be her child. The calmness with which he faced the long surgery ahead impressed her.

After Andy's admission to the hospital, Mardini visited Andy in his room. He and Andy shook hands and started talking. Mardini explained some technicalities and paperwork they had to get out of the way. He presented Andy with the final consent forms to sign. They had spoken together many times previously about the risks and consequences of the surgery, but discussions just before serious operations often carry a stronger urgency than conversations that happen way in advance, when the surgery seems merely a possibility. Mardini asked Andy if he was certain he wanted to undergo the transplant.

"Yes, I'm ready," Andy replied.

"We're going to do the best we can," Mardini said. "Do you have any questions?"

Research fellow Marissa Suchyta was present, and Andy's composure surprised her. "He was so ready for this to happen and had so much trust in the team that he had no hesitation signing those consent forms," she said.

Amer too evaluated Andy. He once again told Andy about the risks and possible complications of the face transplant. They also discussed Andy's CMV mismatch with the donor's tissues and the medications and treatments that could minimize any potential problems. Amer judged that the risk of Andy undergoing anesthesia was acceptable.

Mardini asked Mayo photographer Eric Sheahan to take a portrait of Andy to record what Andy looked like before the face transplant. Sheahan introduced himself and explained his mission. He thought his request made Andy uncomfortable. Andy treated Sheahan kindly, but "there was tension in the room," Sheahan said. Andy did not want to look at the camera, but Sheahan was able to capture images of Andy that showed his high emotions at the time.

Even though the face transplant would not start until the early morning hours of Saturday, the team was notified and ready by midafternoon on Friday. Mardini suggested to Karim Bakri that they use the time remaining to go home and get some sleep. Both men returned home, but neither slept. Bakri and his wife had two small children. That week his mother-in-law was a houseguest. To maintain Andy's privacy and the secrecy of the transplant, Bakri had to hide from her what he would be doing for the next three days. "She thought I was on call, except that I went out Friday night and didn't come back until Monday," he said. He added, smiling: "It was a complicated case, you know."

Bakri did not feel stressed, but he was aware of the high expectations he, Mardini, and the other team members shouldered. They were going into a type of surgery that had never been attempted at Mayo, but their practice on cadavers had led them to believe it could be done successfully. Bakri described his feelings at the time as "not wanting to disappoint, wanting everything to go really smoothly in something that you've never done before." He did not know what was going to happen, and he felt like he was taking a trip to the moon without knowing if he would be able to return to Earth.

Early on Friday, Mardini held a team meeting. The group included Katie Weimer, vice president of 3D Corporation, the company that had provided the three-dimensional models the team used in its rehearsals. Weimer had been involved from the start in the virtual surgical planning aspects of the surgery. "The day has come," Mardini said at the start of the meeting. "We have all put in so much time and effort and thought into this—we could not be more ready." He felt no need to review the operation itself after so many rehearsals in the cadaver lab. Instead, Mardini presented a schedule for breaks to ensure a high-performing team at the transplant's conclusion, when it would be needed most. He asked team members to take breaks when asked, and not do the courteous thing and offer to keep working.

Knowing the transplant surgery was imminent, ophthalmologist Elizabeth Bradley had canceled all her other appointments starting Friday afternoon. After the meeting, Bradley needed stress relief, so she worked out at the on-site fitness center and returned to duty by late afternoon. Mardini let her and other members of the surgical team know that he would handle last-minute preparations and that they should take it easy, sleeping if possible, until later. The operation was still some hours off, and Bradley went home to rest. The call to report in came at 2:00 a.m. Saturday morning, awakening her. She was back at the hospital at 3:00 a.m.

Andy had presented himself for the face transplant in excellent physical condition, and he seemed to Mardini to be at prime readiness. The surgeon estimated that Andy had worked out five or six days per week before the operation in addition to his rigorous outdoor activities on the job. "He was healthy-looking and strong in his mind," Mardini said. "He said he knew we were preparing hard, and he wanted to do the same."

Andy's dad, Reed, was able to travel to Rochester on short notice for the operation (he ended up staying in Rochester for three months after). After booking a hotel room across the street from the hospital, he got lost trying to find Andy's hospital room. It took a while for him to find it, but he did. Just before the transplant began, Reed gave Mardini a handshake and a hug, and Andy told Reed he loved him.

Together, Mardini and Andy moved toward the operating suite, Andy in a wheelchair, Mardini walking alongside.

The timing of the surgery was fortunate. Hundreds of procedures are underway at Saint Marys on a typical weekday. But because it was a weekend, the hospital's operating rooms were quieter than usual. Adding a face transplant to a normal day of surgery would have ratcheted up the complexity. To do this work during a quiet weekend was perfect—an unintentional circumstance that mirrored all the team's weekend rehearsals and preparations in the cadaver lab. Mayo's surgical leadership would have allowed Andy's face transplant to happen anytime, but luck set the stage for a weekend operation.

Once in the suite, Andy lay down on the operating table and felt an intense urge to hold someone's hand. Nursing supervisor

Lori Schacht approached and began rubbing his hand. It was the first time she had met him. After reassuring him, she gently placed an oxygen mask over his face. She would hold his hand again before each of the several follow-up surgeries Andy would have in the months ahead. In a neighboring room, the face of Rudy's brain-dead body, kept functional by machines, was ready for its part in the opening phase of the procedure.

Pieces of equipment ready to go in the operating suite included maxillofacial mandibular plating systems used to attach tissue to bone from KLS Martin, a firm that had worked closely over the years with Mardini on facial reconstruction cases and over the dozens of Saturdays in the cadaver lab; drills and saws; a piezo-electric saw for fine-detail cutting of bone; and imaging equipment.

It would be the first face transplant operation ever performed at Mayo Clinic and the thirty-ninth performed in the world. It involved practitioners from plastic surgery, oculoplastic surgery, transplant nephrology, anesthesia, transplant surgery, trauma critical care medicine and surgery, neurology, radiology, and many other medical specialties. "The most intense, most difficult procedure I've ever seen," summed up surgical tech Kevin Asprey. Elizabeth Bradley remembered standing at the scrub sink thinking, "OK, we're prepared for this. This is the biggest case I'll ever do. This is our World Series."

The goal was to remove and replace Andy's upper and lower jaw, nose, teeth, palate, cheeks, facial muscles, oral mucosa, the skin of the face from under the eyelids to the neck—ear to ear—and some of the salivary glands. Over the next fifty-six hours, about fifty surgeons, nurses, and other surgical staff would work, some but not all taking four-hour breaks, to make the entire intricate procedure happen.

The surgery differed from most operations in many ways—in its length and intensity, the number of people involved, and the essential coordination with the procurement of the donor's face in an adjoining room. Another distinction was the presence of Mayo's photography and video staff and their documentation of the procedure from start to finish. Eric Sheahan, Kevin Ness, John Lemanski, and others, with permissions from Andy and everyone else involved, worked in shifts to visually document the procedures being performed in both Andy's and the donor's suites.

Most critical to the success of the transplant was their documentation of the facial nerve branches and the muscle movement each branch produced when electrically stimulated, in both Andy and the donor. Ness was charged with photographing the nerves after their dissection from both bodies, and then printing the pictures so that Mardini and his team could note on the photograph the function of each nerve. For example, a nerve may be responsible for 80 percent of a smile and 20 percent of an eyelid closure. Andy and the donor each received this intense analysis.

A kindred challenge was locating the nerves once the donor's face was moved to Andy. During Mardini's travels studying face transplants, his friends and other transplant surgeons had generously shared their experiences with him. One face transplant team had trouble with the length of the facial nerve branches when it was time to connect the organ with the patient. Massive swelling that appeared during the face transplant made it nearly impossible to join the cut nerves. Consequently, Mardini planned to procure as much as possible of the nerve branches from the donor, extending all the way to the base of the donor's skull, and to leave Andy with all the nerve length possible. By this plan, when the structures and tissues of the new face were brought to Andy and the bones were connected, Mardini would overlap the donor's nerves with Andy's nerves. Only then, if the surgical team felt certain the donor's nerves matched and overlapped correctly with Andy's, would Andy's existing nerves be cut.

Great care was to be taken with the nerve segments to ensure that Andy's new facial muscles could accurately respond to signals from his brain. If it was done correctly, then when Andy wanted to smile, impulses from his brain would activate the corresponding transplanted facial nerves to correctly curve the mouth upward rather than close the mouth or perform another unintended movement. The same painstaking process would enable Andy to speak, cry, and perform other facial functions correctly. To ensure that all the nerves matched properly between the donor and Andy, Mardini asked Mayo resident Waleed Gibreel, who would later join Mardini's craniofacial team at Mayo, and research fellow Marissa Suchyta to watch and double-check the videos showing the stimulation of the nerves of the donor and patient. Mardini and the team then knew with certainty which nerves to connect from Andy to the donor.

In Andy's suite, Mayo's videographers used an eerily silent overhead video system that they controlled from a console. It had an arm that rose above the surgery and shot straight down. It ran constantly, supplemented by footage from handheld cameras. "We got engaged," Sheahan said. "We made sure the camera was where it needed to be. We didn't let somebody stand in the way, and we spoke up when we needed to take a photo, because we were helping Andy [to] have greater success when we spoke up if something was not right." Sheahan's aggressive methods in the operating room, shooting in the intense quiet, led him to call himself "the surgeon's henchman."

"You weren't just there to capture images," said Kevin Ness. "You engaged yourself in the surgery, so you knew what's going on and you knew when there was a picture needed. And you were right there, and they didn't even have to ask you to take a picture. You just did it."

This photographic diligence was necessary not only to document the face transplant and crucially aid in the surgery but also to preserve what transpired in the surgical suites as a learning aid for surgeons and perhaps face transplants to come. The record of this long weekend for Andy and Mardini in Saint Marys would teach and inspire caregivers far into the future.

~

Shortly before the transplant would begin, Rudy arrived from a hospital in Sioux Falls, South Dakota, where his brain death had been declared. Mayo neurologist Alejandro Rabinstein checked Rudy in, noted the condition of his body, and made sure all went as planned. Rabinstein's goal was to keep Ross's body ventilated and his blood flowing until the procurement of his face and other organs could begin.

A complication arose as soon as Mardini and his procurement team had a chance to examine Rudy. Serious periodontal disease was evident. This was potentially dangerous to Andy because the diseased gum tissue could later introduce pathogens to Andy's immunosuppressed system. How great was the risk? After consulting with prosthodontist Thomas Salinas, Mardini determined the risk was manageable and the procurement could move ahead, with the understanding that Salinas would treat the gum problems soon after the transplant.

In some ways, the removal of donated organs from Rudy's body followed the usual procedures in place for all donors: LifeSource would allocate organs to different medical centers based on the best matches between donors and patients on the list. Each team would then send surgeons to procure the internal organs and ready them for rapid shipment to their intended recipients. In other respects, however, the removal of organs from Rudy's body deviated from the usual plan.

Typically, the procurement process takes place in the same hospital where the donor has been declared brain dead. But in this instance, only Mardini had the expertise to take on the unusual procedure of procuring the donor's face. This meant the donor had to be brought to Rochester. In addition, in this procurement process, the face had to take precedence over the other organs to be donated. While Mardini worked on its removal, the face had to remain fully perfused with blood to keep its tissues usable and healthy during the many hours it took to procure it. And that could happen only if the heart, lungs, and other organs kept doing their work, with the aid of machinery.

Two years before Andy's transplant, LifeSource employees Susan Gunderson and Meg Rogers met with the Mayo team to discuss the forthcoming surgery, which was unprecedented in the Upper Midwest region. They resolved to inform all the solid organ surgical teams in the region that when a face transplant donor was identified, the donor would be transported to Mayo Clinic so that the side-by-side operating suites could work together. Arranging to transport a donor after brain death is not simple. In a process that took over a year, coroners gave approval, solid organ procurement teams agreed to go to Mayo, and everyone on those teams approved a process of waiting for Mardini and his team to finish procuring the face before procurement of other organs began. The various groups' activities had to coordinate smoothly to prevent damage to the organs involved. If organs such as the heart or liver fared poorly, the lives of the recipients could be at risk. Furthermore, damage to other organs during facial tissue procurement could hinder the entire field of face transplantation. "This could absolutely not happen," Mardini said.

Because the procurement of the donor's face was expected to take between twelve and twenty hours, Mayo agreed to place its own solid organ surgeons on standby in case the donor became unstable during the face procurement. If such a problem developed, the standby teams would rush in to take the organs, and Mardini's face transplant team would have to abandon its own procurement.

Mayo transplant surgeons Richard "Rocky" Daly, Julie Heimbach, Charles Rosen, Timucin Taner, and others were ready to take such emergency action if necessary.

Before work began on Rudy's face, Meg Rogers read a statement from the donor's family to the assembled staff. In a minute or so of text, it lovingly told of Ross's love of hunting with his dogs and his best personal qualities. The fifteen to twenty Mayo team members—two or three times more people than Rogers was accustomed to addressing at other procurement operations—maintained a moment of silence. The message from Rudy's family positioned him not just as a source of organs but as a real person. The Mayo team realized as well that Rudy's donation amounted to more than his face; his other organs could save the lives of several other people, and the group had to make every effort to protect all the organs. "What impressed me was that the leadership from Mayo, who had been involved in this process the whole way through, were present in that huddle to be supportive," Rogers said.

Transplant nurse coordinator Lori Ewoldt will never forget what she saw that evening. She watched the transplant team getting ready to start the procurement process, and organ procurement surgeons waiting to take Rudy's stupendous gifts. Ewoldt is not an outwardly emotional person. But this scene overwhelmed her. "Oh, boy," the recollection made Ewoldt exclaim. "Wow. Wow."

In Rudy's suite, Mardini began marking Rudy's face, making the incisions, raising the skin, and methodically locating the facial nerve branches and blood vessels supplying the face. Every nerve branches out like a tree, and the neural paths become more complex as they branch further, into smaller "twigs." Each branch of the pathway is responsible for specific neural functions. Electrically stimulating them revealed their functions, and the team video-recorded the results.

Having finished one side of Rudy's face, Mardini left Bakri and Martinez-Jorge to continue the process on the other side while he moved next door to Andy's suite. There, with the help of Uldis Bite and Basel Sharaf, he initiated a similar process on Andy— marking his face, making the incisions, raising the skin, and mapping the nerves and blood vessels.

Although Bakri was performing part of the procurement, Mardini was the boss. He "made the decisions that I [carried out]," Bakri said. "I'm executing his plan, our plan." Periodically, Mardini called on the phone from the neighboring suite to check on Bakri's progress. Bakri discovered that once the operation got going, he felt no stress. It was even enjoyable. He was looking forward to whatever was coming. "I hate to say it like that, but we enjoy what we do," he said. He was operating in a world he loved.

The concurrent procedures of procuring Rudy's face and preparing Andy to receive it inched forward. Mardini moved from one suite to the other. Two microscopes, one in Andy's suite and one in the donor's, aided this work. For the first time in a face transplant, Mardini and his team were using virtual surgical planning and 3D-printed cutting guides, along with other innovative fitting guides. The surgeons saw with relief that the guides perfectly fit Andy's face. The 3D-printed plastic guides snapped onto the zygomas, the bones around the eyes, to guide where the surgeons would make their cuts to remove Andy's facial tissue. These guides bore slits the precise width of the surgical blades, ensuring that the team made the osteotomies, or incisions, at the proper angle and depth. Having those cutting decisions determined in advance simplified the surgeons' work.

Eventually Mardini reached a decisive point in the surgery. The skin had been lifted off the underlying tissues of Andy's face, the nerves had been identified and mapped for their function, and blood vessels to nourish the transplanted tissues had been identified and dissected out. Up to this point, the incisions would leave permanent scars on Andy but no lasting damage if the surgery had to stop in the event Rudy's body became unstable and solid organ teams had to take action to procure the lifesaving organs. Now Mardini had reached the point of no return. The next steps—cutting Andy's facial nerves and severing Andy's facial bones—would create irreparable damage. At that point only bones and tissue from Rudy's face could give Andy the kind of life he hoped for.

In the donor's suite, Bakri received another call from Mardini: Should Mardini press ahead past the point of no return? Was the donor stable? Was there any possibility the solid organs might be compromised while waiting for the face procurement to be completed? If the donor were to become unstable, solid organs would need to be removed promptly and procurement of the face halted. Mardini needed a definitive answer. For Bakri, this was a satisfying moment. Mardini could have scrubbed out of Andy's suite and decided for himself after examining Rudy, but he relied on Bakri's judgment. "I know he felt at that point that he's got the right partner, he's trained the right guy, that we're all a team, that he's got faith in the team," Bakri said. "It's a big deal for a surgeon to be like me in that situation, and for him to say 'Carry on.'" It was a quick moment, in that nothing really happened, but "emotionally and internally, for me, it was the biggest moment, and we just carried on."

While Mardini finished preparing Andy, Bakri and his group had time on their hands in the donor suite. He decided to ad-lib in a useful way. He opened Rudy's neck and excavated out the carotid artery. The transplant plan had not called for using the carotid to supply blood to the transplanted face, but it is a large vessel and would provide a longer reach to Andy's neck and potentially more blood to the new face than the vessel they had originally planned on using. The team prepared the carotid to immediately deliver blood to the face when it left for the adjoining suite. This took time—which the team had—and hands on deck, which were in short supply at that moment.

Bakri's surgical partner Martinez-Jorge was not in the suite then, so Bakri called upon oculoplastic surgeon Bradley, overseeing the eyelids, to shift gears. She scrubbed in and helped hold the retractors while Bakri extracted the carotid. Never as a surgeon had she been into that part of the human anatomy. It was effort well spent because the team would find the carotid ready to go later in the transplant. "That really made a difference. It helped everyone sleep better" later, Bakri said. Before the transplant was over, Bradley would prove to be a valuable team member with a magnificent spirit, Mardini realized.

It took more than twenty hours—five hours longer than expected—to excise Rudy's facial skin, muscles, nerves, and bones. Returning to Rudy's suite to finish the final stages of the procurement, Mardini focused his attention on disimpacting the face—separating the bones of the face from the skull after the cuts were performed on the upper and lower jaws and all other parts of the operation were complete. Finally, a critical moment arrived. Rudy's facial organ was completely separated from his body, ready to be flushed with heparin (a blood anticoagulant) and saline before being moved to Andy's suite. Although seeing the full detachment of the donor's face felt surreal to everyone in the room, there was no time for emotion. The adrenaline-fueled intensity of all that lay ahead did not allow the participants to dwell on the moment.

The other surgeons engaged by LifeSource, there to procure the internal organs available for donation, appeared to be "circling around" with their containers for organs, according to one person present. Mayo Clinic's Transplant Center director, Brooks Edwards, remembers them sitting and eating doughnuts, worried about the patients already on operating tables in other cities, "waiting for the liver, waiting for the lungs." Many people's lives were on hold and on the line. These physicians were not used to waiting.

Inside the surgical suites, Mardini sensed the heat of their restlessness and worry. Feeling compelled to calm their fears, Mardini left Rudy's suite and told the waiting surgeons he understood the importance of their efforts to obtain the other organs. He acknowledged holding up their work. For three years, he let them know, Mardini and his team had practiced the procurement of the donor's face, and Andy was past the point of no return in the neighboring surgical suite. Andy's face had been removed, and he must have the donor's face. Mardini "was very professional but wanted to make sure everyone was heard and that he addressed any questions and welcomed input," Rogers said. "It was phenomenal."

Edwards delicately suggested to Mardini that he take no more than another two hours to complete procurement of the face. "I felt a little uncomfortable, as a non-surgeon, to tell him to finish up the operation," Edwards admits, but everybody was concerned about losing the donor. Mardini ended up needing a little more than the two hours Edwards offered. During that time, Edwards summoned to the hospital Mayo cardiac surgeon Rocky Daly to talk with the waiting surgeons and help relieve their stress. "Rocky's presence made the biggest difference," Mardini said, remembering that Daly told him, "You are doing great—keep doing what you are doing, and I will deal with the rest." It was a moment Mardini never forgot and will forever appreciate.

As soon as Mardini completed the removal of Rudy's face, solid organ teams joined the operation and procured Rudy's kidneys, pancreas, liver, lungs, and heart after Rogers of LifeSource authorized the clamping of Rudy's aorta, halting the blood flow. The surgeons accomplished those procurements in a complexly choreographed free-for-all.

But the work on the donor was not yet complete, even after all his organs designated for donation had been removed. Anaplastologists Gillian Duncan and Michaela Calhoun—medical artists on the team who specialized in facial prosthetics—were busy giving

Rudy's face creative attention. Mardini had recruited this talented pair, who had previously worked with his team in the Saturday cadaver lab sessions, hoping they could accomplish something completely new: to use their skills and materials to build a prosthetic face for Rudy that would look as real as the prosthetics they crafted for living patients. The goal was to give completeness and dignity to Rudy's body when it left the operating room, and to allow for an open-casket funeral if that was what the family wished. Using a moulage, or clay mold, of Rudy's face, Duncan and Calhoun spent about ninety minutes with Gibreel to fit and sew the mask to the area where Rudy's face had been.

Later, Meg Rogers witnessed the amazement of the funeral director collecting Rudy's body when he saw the realistic mask. "He thought he had the wrong patient because he believed this was supposed to be the face donor, and the body had a lifelike face," she said. The funeral home director notified Lilly Ross, Rudy's widow, of the success of Duncan and Calhoun's mask. Lilly, accompanied by Rudy's mother, viewed Rudy's body at the funeral home and was struck by the care and respectfulness that the preparation of the mask communicated about how Rudy had been treated. In a scene that mixed sadness and joy, Lilly and Rudy's mother were able to see Rudy's face one last time.

In Andy's surgical suite, a difficulty arose. Andy began the transplant with a metal plate in his jaw from his earlier reconstruction operations. Now the surgical team was having trouble cutting through it with the available drill bits. Despite the team's practice in the cadaver lab, this unexpected roadblock complicated the real-life application of the long-practiced techniques. "We went through a lot of different equipment trying to get that [plate] off," Schacht said. It was critical to remove it without damaging the surrounding bones because Andy's jaw structure would later have to meld cleanly with the donor's. "If that fractured, that was going to be a big, big deal," remembered Bradley. Using too much torque "would fracture the whole thing, and the plate had been in there long enough to get bone ingrowth—it was just like concrete."

Bite asked for every diamond burr, an expensive drill part, that the hospital had in stock. There were twenty-five available, and Bite wanted all of them at hand, just in case. Three screws of the plate proved especially difficult to remove, but Bite and Sharaf eventually succeeded in extracting them without damage to the jaw.

In a room near Andy's operating suite, the team had set up a lounge of sorts filled with blankets and furniture that people could use for breaks and naps. "I think I slept there for about an hour throughout the whole thing," said Suchyta, who worked as a runner for team members needing supplies and tissue samples delivered to the pathology lab. "It was a once-in-a-lifetime experience, which is why I didn't want to sleep," Suchyta said. One of the surgeons used his break as an opportunity to apply Bengay to his sore neck.

In the first twenty-four hours of Andy's surgery, Mardini and the team had successfully removed the facial structures that needed to go. "You really can't go back after that," Suchyta remembered. "Everyone held their breath and said, 'OK, here we go.'" The rest of the surgery, another thirty-two hours, would focus on making Rudy Ross's face an integral part of Andy's body.

# Chapter 9

# Danger and Joy

———

More than twenty hours after the procurement began, Mardini, working with Karim Bakri and Jorys Martinez-Jorge, completed the removal of Rudy's face—a complex network of skin, nerves, blood vessels, bone, and muscle. Surgical tech Kevin Asprey remembered the moment: "Now we knew that this was something that we had a great opportunity to present to Andy and change his life in a [profound] way."

For research fellow Marissa Suchyta, this instant marked her personal point of no return. "When the face was procured from the donor, and that was successful, and they had the face on the table—that was a moment when I felt that now we had to move forward, and all this was working," she said.

Using photos and videos taken during the operations in the two separate suites, the team matched each of the countless nerve branches and blood vessels—some barely visible to the naked eye—on Andy's old face with the corresponding pathways on Rudy's face. The sutures they used were likewise invisible except under a microscope. This critical process was tedious and delicate, and it required precision, skill, and time. Everyone hoped the result would be successful nourishment of the new tissues and functional facial movements and sensations. When Andy wanted to smile, eat, or kiss—all the things he had longed to do for years following his facial reconstruction—he should soon be able to do just that.

The surgical team rotated in and out of Andy's operating room. Some took breaks on the beds set up in the neighboring room. Others, like Mardini, barely stopped working. He had reached the point of such deep tiredness that he did not feel tired anymore. Food ordered from nearby restaurants kept the team going. Nurse coordinator Lori Ewoldt made sure everyone was fully fed and hydrated. Nurses and physicians with administrative roles, like Ewoldt, Hatem Amer, and Brooks Edwards, do not normally appear at surgeries, but in this case they did to make sure all was going well and to serve in any way they could. Their presence inspired the others.

Mardini and Bakri began the exacting task of joining the transplanted facial blood vessels to Andy's circulatory system. They sutured an artery and then a vein in an alternating process, providing for the inflow and outflow of blood to the various areas of the face. Studies of previous face transplant procedures showed that connecting the facial artery on one side only could be enough to supply the entire face, including bones. Mardini and Bakri, however, decided to make the blood vessel connections on both sides, to ensure reliable and sufficient flow and provide a backup.

Mardini went first, working on a narrow vessel. He enjoyed working on small vessels, and his skills allowed him to connect them without difficulty. Bakri did the next, a large vessel. He preferred working on the big ones that provided ample flow. Together they connected artery and vein, and then another pair. Over several hours, this work seemed to progress smoothly. When Mardini unclamped the first artery, the face turned pink immediately.

Success! With unimpeded blood circulating in the face, the relief in the operating room was enormous. It was hardly believable that the procedure had come this far without any serious complications.

With the new face already starting to work for Andy, Bakri turned to his colleague and suggested Mardini take a much-needed break. Mardini agreed and left the operating room as Bakri continued making vascular connections. After about a half hour, "I noticed in my peripheral vision that the face was looking pale," Bakri said. "That's not a good sign." The blood flow had slowed or ceased, and with alarm Bakri called Mardini back into the operating room. Bakri believed Andy's blood flow had possibly kinked or clotted after Bakri turned the patient's head to better access the vessels he was then connecting.

Mardini agreed that Bakri should remove some of the sutures in one vessel Mardini had earlier worked on, to get a look inside. "Normally, in situations of blockage we cut out the whole section and redo the whole thing, especially if there was a technical error and you did it wrong the first time. I knew that wasn't the case—I had watched every stitch go in," Bakri said.

Bakri opened one or two sutures in the blood vessel and fished out a clot. "We fixed it; it was fine," Bakri said. Relieved, he left on a short break. Several hours later, when everything in the operating room had been going well for a long time and Bakri was taking one of a couple of forty-five-minute naps he would take during the entire weekend, he received a page. He learned that the transplant had taken a bad turn, and now Mardini needed him immediately. This was ominous. "There's nothing good about being woken up when he knows you're tired," Bakri said.

When Bakri returned to the surgical suite, Mardini was sitting at the microscope, which puzzled Bakri because hours earlier they had completed work on the blood vessels that needed microscopic examination. Then Bakri looked at Andy's face. "It was whiter than any white I've seen," he said. Edwards, present in the room, called this shade of white "dead-looking." Bakri later described it as "ice white, a weird look, scary for a surgeon, scary." Mardini and Bakri did not know the reason behind this potentially catastrophic development. Due to an unknown cause, something was now keeping the transplanted tissues from receiving a sufficient flow of blood. Without adequate blood supply, Andy's new tissues would die. Three years of practice on cadavers had not prepared them for this crisis.

The room fell silent. Apprehensively, the team gathered around Mardini, just watching. "It was an awful, awful, awful moment," Bakri said. Mardini asked the anesthesiologist to report Andy's blood pressure and questioned whether any medication had been administered that might cause blood clotting or constriction of the vessels. But Andy had received no such medication. Bakri had never seen Mardini so miserable. "I could see him just dying inside, and I didn't know anything about what was going on," he recalled. That moment, Mardini later said in his understated way, "was not very comfortable."

Mardini refused to panic, but his face showed his alarm. "Dr. Mardini's face turned as white as the donor face at that point," Suchyta remembered. "It felt like an eternity." Mardini later mentioned that he had not had the option of panicking. He was responsible for the success of this transplant, and he had to summon all his reserves of skill and stamina to make it work. If the lack of blood flow to the face could not be resolved, the team would have to remove the donor face and cover Andy's facial opening with muscle and skin flaps they would take from other parts of his body. All that remained of Andy's old and reconstructed facial tissue were eyeballs, tongue, and neck vessels—and literally nothing else. The face transplant would have failed, leaving Andy with a destroyed face. The flap coverage might help Andy survive the experience, although that was not guaranteed. It would have been the worst possible outcome of the surgery, other than Andy's death.

Bakri asked if Mardini wanted him to scrub in. In a steady and calm voice, Mardini said yes. Both surgeons knew that if they could not get the transplanted face to circulate blood here on the operating table, their situation was dire. They began reopening blood vessels one by one. They saw no clots, nothing unusual—the vessels looked perfect. The surgeons speculated that maybe the entire network of blood vessels circulating the face was going into spasm for unknown reasons. "Just like if the power goes out in your whole house, it's probably not one little fuse somewhere, there's probably something bigger happening," Bakri reasoned.

Mardini called Amer back into the room. "Could this be a massive episode of rejection?" Mardini asked. Rejection could cause the vessels in the donor face to become inflamed and clogged. Amer considered the question. He told Mardini it was unlikely that rejection was causing the problem. Tests had showed that Andy and Rudy, while not completely compatible immunologically, had not shown any previous exposure to each other's antigens and were not immunologically primed against each other. Because there were no pre-formed antibodies, such a hyperacute rejection was unlikely.

Mardini and Bakri together followed a mental checklist of what to do. At the top of the list was clamping and removing a small segment around the arterial connection that could be the location of the problem. Essentially, they would redo the connection, or anastomosis, they had previously performed—even though they had not found a clot when they had partially opened that vessel before. Mardini and Bakri were seasoned reconstructive microsurgeons who often dealt with vascular problems of this kind in their normal practice. Usually, this type of scenario does not end up with a good outcome. This was a face transplant, though, further elevating the stakes. Bakri remembers thinking, "Let's just do it and see—it's got to work." They spent twenty anguished minutes redoing the connective work, not allowing themselves to be tortured by the possibility of disaster.

All around them, staff photographers and videographers continued documenting their work. The overhead camera silently captured Bakri's and Mardini's determined efforts. Staff photographer Kevin Ness took a portrait of Mardini during these moments. "He had such an intense look. . . . You can just see the seriousness and the intensity of his eyes," said Ness, convinced he would remember this image for the rest of his career.

When Mardini and Bakri reopened the vessel, they were able to view through its interior space from one end to the other. There was nothing wrong with the vessel. "It looked pristine," Mardini said. Why would there be no blood flow when the blood supply from Andy's neck vessels was strong and there was no clotting? This was what the surgeons needed to figure out.

At this intense moment, Martinez-Jorge, a calm and thoughtful surgeon, leaned toward Mardini and whispered into his ear a few words that changed the course of the face transplant. Martinez-Jorge explained that while Mardini had earlier been out of the room, retractors had been placed to gain exposure to Andy's lower jaw. Martinez-Jorge wondered if that could have contributed to the problem. Mardini and Bakri thought through this suggestion and speculated whether the use of the retractors might have caused the facial artery's muscles to spasm or constrict, blocking the flow of blood. To investigate the possibility, Mardini put his eyes to the microscope and, with extreme caution, proceeded to strip through the outer layer of the facial artery, beginning at the point of connection with Andy's artery and going all the way back into the transplant tissue. Any mistake in this procedure would leave holes in the artery, a challenge to fix. A few centimeters into the transplanted facial tissue, beyond any place that was exposed to the outside world, Mardini found a clear point of spasm in the facial artery. Mardini released the constricted layer, and blood immediately resumed flowing to the transplanted face.

"The whole thing went pink again," Bakri said, "and oh my God, that sends shivers down [my back] remembering that." The room filled with joy.

"I've never seen Dr. Mardini look so relieved," Suchyta said.

During the operation, Mardini grabbed three opportunities to make brief phone calls to his wife, Rawan. The final call came soon after this gut-wrenching and dangerous episode. "He was crying," Rawan later remembered. "I asked him what was wrong. He said, 'We almost lost the patient.' I put my hand over my mouth and asked, 'What happened?' He said, 'I just remembered every single detail of what I learned in Taiwan, and we were able to make it work.' . . . It still gives me goose bumps when I talk about it."

The surgical work continued. Some parts of the procedure, long practiced in the lab, had to be postponed. Before the surgery, Bradley, the team's oculoplastic surgeon, had been present in every practice session in the cadaver lab, tirelessly rehearsing the process of connecting the eyelid drainage system from donor to recipient. This would allow tears from Andy's eyelids to flow to the transplanted nose on both sides of the face. As the transplant team neared the end of the surgery, however, Bradley and Mardini decided to hold off on placing the bone grafts necessary for the drainage system. Because of all the swelling expected after surgery, both physicians were concerned that the grafts would constrict the space around the eyeballs and cause Andy blindness.

Finally, everything was in place, with blood vessels, nerve fibers, and all tissue connected. It looked like a perfect match—so much so that it almost felt eerie to some in the room. The odds of accomplishing that degree of match while finding a donor whose immune profile so closely aligned with Andy's seemed unbelievable.

Soon Mardini, sitting on a stool behind Andy's head, set a blue towel over Andy's new and fully attached face. With a palm on each side of the face, he squeezed for nearly ten minutes, slowly diminishing the swelling within the tissues. By using this procedure to reduce swelling, Mardini enabled the skin to close and heal more precisely.

Once the skin was thus closed, the face transplant procedure was over. An image shot by the photo crew shows Mardini, drained and tired but radiating joy. In the time since the operation started, he had grown a beard. There had been no needles lost, no miscounts of equipment, and no mistakes. It was now 8:00 a.m. on the morning of Monday, June 13, 2016.

After completing the transplant, Mardini spoke through his exhaustion to call the transplant "a miracle." Nine surgeons and some forty operating room staff had pulled it off. They felt excited and elated. Adrenaline had propelled them during the long shifts. Lori Schacht considered it the most amazing surgery she had experienced over a long career. Long and fascinating liver transplants she had worked on did not rival it.

The team had worked carefully to make sure no unauthorized people knew about Andy's transplant. There was a security presence inside the hospital, and the staff knew to keep the transplant confidential. Any slip might mean the release of a photo of Andy—a violation of his privacy that could harm his dignity as a recovering patient. The team wanted the release of any image of Andy and his new face to happen only when he was ready, when his face looked like any other face.

After leaving the operating room, Bakri bumped into a colleague who had taken on a reconstructive surgery that Bakri had had to forgo over the long weekend. That colleague was almost in tears, deeply moved by the magnitude of the treatment the transplant team had given Andy.

# Chapter 10

# Awakening

———

A ndy's face transplant had taken two and a half days.
The day the surgery was completed, June 13, was Reed's
birthday. Reed had driven to Rochester and arrived
at Saint Marys just a couple of hours before Andy's transplant
began. Seeing Andy calmly waiting for the procedure, Reed had
asked, "How are you not freaking out?" Andy explained that he
felt peace of mind, and he had confidence in his medical team,
having been fully prepared by Mayo staff over the previous
three years.

The surgery had made Reed nervous. Afterward, he spoke with
Danielle Peabody Reuss, a Mayo social worker, and admitted that
he understood little of the medical discussions in which he had
participated. But it was clear to him that the surgical and ICU
teams were giving Andy thorough and attentive care. "It's a well-
oiled machine," he told Reuss. He expected the worst—a gravely
damaged patient—when Andy emerged from the transplant, but

he felt relieved and pleasantly surprised by Andy's appearance in the ICU.

Andy was heavily sedated for several days after the face transplant. The team had planned to keep him sedated for a day or so after the operation to be certain he would be stable when he awoke. But "as soon as we lightened the sedation, his blood pressure went up to the 170s and 180s, systolic, which is unusual for a young patient who is healthy," Mardini said. Mardini worried that the high blood pressure could cause a rupture of Andy's blood vessels or damage the transplanted tissue. Persistent redness in the facial skin also raised concerns about tissue rejection. The team eventually concluded that vessels were not yet properly regulating blood flow and that it would be better to keep Andy sedated a while longer.

When Andy arrived in the ICU, he needed ventilator support to breathe and required a complex medication regimen. He was at risk for severe complications, including catastrophic bleeding from reattached blood vessels, blood pressure instability, blood clotting, infection, and inflammation that could injure his kidneys, lungs, or other organs. He was placed on a lifetime immunosuppression regimen with three medications, similar to those used for kidney or heart transplant patients. Facial redness or swelling could indicate tissue rejection, and severe rejection could lead to the death of the facial tissue. Another risk was that his suppressed immune system would be unable to fight off opportunistic infections.

Christopher Arendt, the pharmacist on Andy's transplant team, compared the risks of Andy's situation to making copies of copies on a photocopier. "[The original image] degrades, right?" he said. "Our cells are getting copies made of them perpetually, and we make copies of our copies of our copies, and eventually we crank out a bad copy. Our immune system is responsible for finding that bad copy." Suppression of the immune system allows the bad copy of a cell to pass unnoticed and eventually cause problems, such as an increased risk of skin cancer or kidney damage. The advantage of immunosuppressants is that they help a person tolerate transplanted tissue. The disadvantage is that the medications have side effects that can shorten life span. "The assumption is when people go on immunosuppression, if they don't need it for an organ that prolongs their life, we are likely shortening their life span," Amer said.

To guard against the previously identified risk of cytomegalovirus infection from the donor's tissues, Andy also received the antiviral medication valganciclovir. Under Razonable's guidance, the team carefully monitored Andy's immune system for signs of improvement in his ability to fight off infection. Once Andy's immune system recovered sufficiently from the intense immunosuppression during the transplant procedure, they stopped the antiviral medication and Andy was monitored very closely for appearance of CMV. When the virus did appear and Andy's immune system had a chance to "see" it, the valganciclovir was quickly resumed and the virus suppressed. This brief exposure to CMV allowed Andy's immune system to develop antibodies against the virus that would protect him even when he was no longer on the antiviral medication. All of this happened without Andy experiencing any symptoms—a major feat of immunological medicine.

Because of the complexity of Andy's case, the lead physicians divided responsibilities for his care: Mardini and his team looked after Andy's surgical concerns, Amer oversaw the patient's drug regimen, and Jowsey-Gregoire managed his psychiatric needs. They frequently communicated with each other and jointly made hospital rounds to visit Andy at least twice per day, despite having many responsibilities to other patients. Andy's recovery required an intense and remarkable degree of teamwork from the staff to keep him out of peril. To protect Andy's privacy, only staff members with a specific need to see him were given access to Andy's room. All told, hundreds of Mayo employees contributed to Andy's recovery.

The day after the completion of the transplant, Andy's facial graft appeared stable. The perfusion of blood to the face looked excellent. Andy also carried an additional piece of transplanted tissue—a portion grafted from Rudy's left leg to Andy's groin—known as a sentinel flap, which would serve as an area for protocol biopsies (sparing his face) and for early detection of any tissue rejection. It appeared as a large bulge, as it should. Over the next several days, his recovery went as expected. When the staff inspected Andy's oral cavity, all sutures were intact, and the transplanted tissues in his mouth appeared stable. To prevent bedsores, nurses turned his body every two hours.

Just before the surgery, Andy had received a tracheostomy, an opening directly to his windpipe, and an endotracheal tube that allowed him to breathe without the use of his mouth or nose while the procedure took place. Once Andy awakened after the operation, he would receive a tracheostomy collar to use with the tube. As the muscles of his mouth and throat gained strength, he would be able to better control his own breathing and eventually would no longer need the tracheostomy collar.

By the third day following the surgery, Andy's blood pressure was improving and the team felt it was safe to reduce Andy's sedation. It took another several days for him to wake up. On the sixth day, he gained consciousness in room 582 of the Saint Marys intensive care unit. He dimly saw Reed sitting in the room. Andy made a motion with his arm and went back to sleep. Later, Reed asked Andy what he remembered of that first awakening. Andy recalled trying to talk and being unable to make a sound or express himself in any way. He wanted to tell his dad: "In two more weeks this trach is coming out, and we're going home." It was a brain-fogged and inaccurate prediction, as Andy's stay in the hospital's ICU would last another four weeks.

When the staff became aware that Andy had acknowledged the presence of Reed in his hospital room, they noted that Andy also was able to move his arms and legs, follow other commands, open and close his eyes and jaw, and shake his head in answer to questions about pain and discomfort. His graft and skin tone still looked excellent. The facial skin appeared to redden and lighten in concert with changes in his blood pressure.

As Andy recovered, his team worked to maintain his privacy. Before the transplant, Mayo's communications staff had urged Andy to take control of the release of information about his surgery. He had also received media training, the first time former communications manager Ginger Plumbo could remember a patient receiving such preparation.

Andy, who had lived reclusively before the transplant, wanted no interviews or sharing of his story before he was ready. He had told as few people as possible about his forthcoming procedure. His family kept the secret as well. Several security workers were tasked with keeping away any journalists or outsiders who might have heard rumors of the face transplant, with one security staff member always planted outside his door. "We were really worried about press sneaking in," said transplant center administrator Lori Ewoldt, and for a time she considered using hats of a particular color to identify those with official access to the patient.

At one point, a drone was spotted hovering outside the window of a room near Andy's. Worried that it might have a camera, the staff called Mayo's security team. Rochester police soon traced the drone to a man in his twenties operating it from a location heavily populated by physicians, called Pill Hill. Recently relocated to Rochester, the man was using the drone to shoot a video showing off his new hometown, which he intended to send to his girlfriend. He knew nothing of Andy or his surgery, and the police gave him the scare of his life. Soon after, the windows of Andy's room were curtained.

Meanwhile, Mayo started reporting Andy's story using its own writers and photographers. It would hold on to these words and images until later, when Andy decided what, if anything, he wanted to do with them.

~

A week after the surgery ended, Andy was showing increasing signs of consciousness. Although still drowsy even after being off sedation medications for a few days, and only occasionally opening his eyes, he communicated with Reed, who remained "easygoing and in high spirits," social worker Reuss observed.

Reed's steadfast presence in Andy's room brought many benefits. It helped orient him even during periods of drowsiness and confusion. Andy felt happy every time he opened his eyes and saw his father. Their conversations—with Andy's part accomplished through head motions and hand gestures—stimulated Andy and speeded his recovery. He frequently reached for Reed and staff to hold hands, and he felt calmed by assurances spoken in a soft voice and by gentle massage of his hands and arms.

Andy's room lacked mirrors, his cellphone was in safekeeping, and he had no idea what his new face looked like. When Amer examined Andy's face, he found some expected swelling but judged Andy's recovery to be proceeding entirely satisfactorily.

Two weeks after the surgery, Reed began considering when he could leave Andy's bedside to make a quick break for home. The social worker said that although Reed's presence had been essential when Andy was regaining consciousness, it now was not as important for Reed to be always present. Andy gave his agreement with a wave of his arm. Even so, Reed was reluctant to leave, and he remained with Andy for many more weeks.

Psychiatrist Jowsey-Gregoire had her first post-transplant interview with Andy on June 22. Squeezing her hand, he communicated that he did not feel frightened. He was still unable to write to express his thoughts. The next day, however, he had made gains in his recovery. When social worker Reuss came for a visit, Andy was in a chair, reclining, and fully awake, watching sports on TV. He indicated to Reuss that earlier he had stood upright and walked a few steps. He used his two fingers to demonstrate a walking motion. Then he reached for a whiteboard and scrawled out a few words, but his writing was illegible and Reuss could not read what he had written.

Early on in his efforts to communicate using the whiteboard, Andy frequently grew frustrated. Shaky from anti-rejection medication and still recovering from his major surgery, he could not control his hand. "My handwriting was absolutely horrible, and nobody could read what I was writing," he said later. The staff tried in vain to understand him, making wild guesses. "Then I'd try to rewrite it, and they wouldn't get it."

With time Andy grew more proficient at writing, but the mental effort was exhausting. Short walks wore him out, too. He rated his mood at 5 on a 10-point scale, adding that fatigue was dragging down his spirits. He said he was not yet interested in looking at his face and wanted to follow Mardini's advice to wait until the swelling diminished. Andy said he did not feel anxious about his appearance. Nonetheless, Jowsey-Gregoire reminded him of the benefits he had gained from the exposure therapy he underwent when he was getting used to his reconstructed face nine years earlier.

In a meeting with Mardini, Jowsey-Gregoire raised the possibility of slowly reintroducing Andy to contact with the outside world. They knew Andy had to remain in the hospital to protect his privacy and to continue his recovery, but without more stimulation, there was a possibility that his mental health might deteriorate. The physicians asked Andy what he would like to do. He mentioned spending time outdoors and riding a bicycle. Building a model airplane would be fun, too. He said he liked dogs, so they promised to investigate the possibility of bringing in a therapy dog. Later Reuss asked if, given his experience as an electrician, Andy would be interested in touring the power station that served the hospital. He nodded enthusiastically.

Meanwhile, Andy frequently walked around the ward. He was required to wear a mask to prevent airborne infection, to have a staff escort, and to be followed at a distance by a security detail. It was quite the retinue. Despite pain in his jaw, Andy was determined to rebuild his strength. He participated in physical therapy and was recovering well.

On June 30, he felt a game changer—a tingling sensation in his nose, possibly caused by stimulation at the nerve ending where Andy's nerve and the donor's nerve were connected. It was perhaps a sign that nerve regeneration was beginning, and it lifted his mood. He was looking forward to riding a stationary bicycle and watching Rochester's upcoming Independence Day fireworks show. He told his physicians that he believed he was regaining his mental sharpness, with less confusion fogging his mind.

That day he and Reed went downstairs and sat together in an outdoor courtyard, accompanied by a nurse. Out in the sun for the first time, Andy was able to speak to his father in short sentences despite still lacking the ability to move his mouth. His surgical mask muffled his speech, yet he was understandable. The excursion, however, was brief. The elevator descent had given Andy an upset stomach, and he tired quickly in the summer humidity.

Over the July 4 holiday, Andy's brother, Ronald, and Ronald's girlfriend came for a visit. It was good to be together, and the hospital's seventh-floor library offered them an excellent view of the fireworks.

Starting in July, many of the lines draining fluid from Andy's face were removed as the swelling decreased and healing progressed. Feeling better, he began communicating through a combination of gesturing, writing, and speaking. He told his social worker that he disliked the constant attention he was receiving from staff, as well as all "the poking and prodding." His frustration undoubtedly arose from his transformation from a healthy and active young man before his face transplant to a hospitalized patient with very little independence.

Andy now felt ready to have a look at his face. He had been bugging Mardini about it for days. "Come on, man, let's just do it," he begged the surgeon. "Let's just get it over with." Mardini continued to ask for patience while the swelling subsided. A week or so earlier, Reed had assured Andy, "I'm telling you, you're going to be happy with what you see," which excited him. "I can't wait," he wrote on the whiteboard. The staff's comments that he looked good only fueled his curiosity. He often gently touched his new face, encouraged by what his fingers told him.

The mirror, however, was going to show Andy a face that wasn't the original Andy, or even the reconstructed Andy. A different face would look back at him. It could be a real shock. Was this truly the best time in Andy's recovery to experience that? His medical team had debated the question for a long time. It was finally Mardini who decided the time was right. He set a date for the big reveal. Reed, Ronald, Ronald's girlfriend, all of Andy's main physicians, a representative of LifeSource, and many from the nursing staff were invited to attend.

The day of the reveal arrived, as dramatic as the unveiling of a public statue. Andy felt what he called "pure excitement." Jowsey-Gregoire, who had been preparing Andy for this event on an almost daily basis, reminded him of his resiliency and the many steps he had taken in his long medical and personal journey. This would be another step. Then someone handed Andy a mirror.

Andy gazed at the image of himself. This new face—still swollen and inflamed, and just barely functional—had once belonged to another human being. The jaw, cheeks, mouth, chin, and teeth he saw in the mirror were not those he had been born with, but there was no denying that his own eyes looked back at him from behind it. Mayo pharmacist Christopher Arendt, who was present, saw happiness and acceptance register on Andy's face. He could imagine Andy letting go of his past and glimpsing what his new life would mean. Reed, deeply moved, later described the moment as "a real tearful, hard-to-hold-back time . . . beyond our wildest dreams." Excitement, anxiety, and apprehension filled the room.

Overcome by emotion, Andy scrawled on his whiteboard: "Far exceeded my expectations." Mardini read this reaction aloud to everyone present in the room. Mardini said in a voice choked by sentiment, "You don't know how happy that makes us feel." Ophthalmologist Elizabeth Bradley, standing in a corner of the crowded room, remembered the unsteadiness of Mardini's voice as he spoke. Everyone was in tears. The moment was unforgettable to those present, most of all Andy. "Once you lose something that you've had forever, you know what it's like not to have it," Andy later told a reporter. "And once you get a second chance to have it back, you never forget it." Despite the drama of the day, Andy's medical transcript recorded the landmark event in a single anticlimactic sentence: "Facial reveal went well and patient very pleased with postoperative outcome."

Andy told Mardini that for the ten years between his injury and the face transplant, he had always seen himself with his original face in his dreams. However, shortly after seeing his transplanted face, he began seeing his new appearance in his dreams. He was already integrating his new face into his sense of self and accepting it as his own.

Bradley, recalling the moment later, noted that when she thinks about Andy, the face she remembers as always belonging to him is the one he acquired through transplant. "Not only does he accept his face," she said, "but we've accepted [it], and that happened very quickly. We accepted that it was his new face, and the memory of the old face is almost gone."

Reed said Andy "would have been smiling from ear to ear" if he had been able to do so. That time would come. In fact, despite the strong emotions of the moment, Andy's expressions were frozen and unrevealing because he still lacked facial movement. Everyone's faces were full of emotion except his. But Andy's eyes hinted at his strong feelings, and the others in the room may have read in them what they imagined he was feeling.

Andy confided to his dad that his new face was better than anything he had thought possible. Having so many people present, with video cameras running, was uncomfortable, but once everyone left him by himself Andy could study his face at leisure. He looked at the suture lines crisscrossing his face, the nasal trumpets that kept open his breathing passages, and his saggy and swollen eyes. He wondered: "When that goes away, what's that going to look like? Hey, I'm a pretty good-looking guy, you know?" Until this time, Andy had not really believed the staff and his family when they told him how good he looked, but now he could see himself and enjoy it.

On that same day, Andy began speech therapy with speech therapists Jack Thomas and Heather Clark. After the transplant surgery, Andy's ability to speak worsened. His original injury had tethered his tongue, and previous facial reconstructive surgeries had adjusted his oral cavity to help him speak and swallow. With his new face, however, the oral cavity was a different size, and his tongue no longer reached the roof of his mouth, making his speech muffled-sounding and difficult to understand. After the transplant, prostho-dontist Thomas Salinas created a retainer-style device to lower the roof of Andy's mouth so his tongue could make contact. This and speech therapy improved his speech until Mardini could perform a follow-up surgery to release his tongue from its tethered position.

Directed by the therapists, Andy practiced non-speech move-ments to stretch and strengthen his mouth, jaw, and tongue. He also tried making exaggerated vocal sounds and prolonged pronunciation of vowels. His lips were not yet in control enough to form such letter sounds as *B, P, M,* and *W.* (The same lack of control over his lips still made it difficult for Andy to eat.) Soft-spoken to begin with, Andy had to learn a new way of speaking. Nearly shouting, Thomas announced, "You've got to talk like this!" Andy had to match his volume, and sometimes nurses peeked in, alarmed at the noise. But his speech improved quickly.

Four weeks after his face transplant, Andy moved out of the ICU and into a seventh-floor room in the hospital. His recovery was likely proceeding so quickly because he was young, healthy, and fit. Andy hoped he would feel less restricted in the new room, with greater access to activities unrelated to his treatment. A surprise awaited him. A group of nurses wanted to give him a tour—along with another organ transplant patient—of the Mayo One helicopter and hangar up on the roof. Andy accepted with delight. "Andy appeared calm and very attentive to the flight nurses' presentation and tour," social worker Reuss wrote. "He was glad to stay a little longer in order to have the opportunity to see a helicopter arrive and land with a patient. Staff took tremendous care to allow him a good view and make him feel comfortable. He shook hands vigorously with many of them at the conclusion of the tour."

Relearning to take food and drink through his mouth was a difficult part of Andy's recovery. At first, when the medical staff urged him to try, Andy resisted. He did not think he was ready to attempt this. He reluctantly agreed to begin with sips of water, under the eye of an imaging machine that monitored the path of liquid through his mouth. Wearing a bib, he initially dribbled water everywhere, but eventually he gained some mastery of the drinking process.

The staff next proposed a trial with applesauce, but Andy was not optimistic. "I told them flat-out no," he said. Despite his initial resistance, he agreed to go through with it even though he felt the outcome would be hopeless. Assured that eating applesauce would not be as bad as he expected, he tried. To his surprise, he found he could move parts of his mouth and feel sensation beneath his cheekbone.

When he told Mardini of this progress, the plastic surgeon looked surprised, too. Mardini had expected sensation to come later. "He comes over, and he starts tapping on my cheekbone," Andy said. That area of Andy's face "lit up a bit," and it made Andy happy. Some of the nerves were firing. Mardini encouraged his patient to try this tapping and touching on his own. Andy's fingers tentatively approached his nose. "I can do that?" he asked. The centering of the nose on his face amazed Andy—his prosthetic nose had been off-center, and it would take him time to get used to having a nose in the right spot.

As Andy regained feeling in his face, he worked with neurologist Beth Robertson to map out the growing areas of sensation. Prior to this, Robertson had worked with Mardini and his medical team, focusing on facial nerve problems and treating facial paralysis and reanimation. With Andy, she used pins to prick his face and plotted out what he felt. Finding the sites Andy could feel for the first time was fascinating for her. It inspired in her a level of professional awe. Years earlier, during her training in neurology, she had learned there was little physicians could do to treat patients with Bell's palsy and other types of facial paralysis and numbness. However, she observed a new standard in Andy's recovery. For the most part, Andy regained sensation starting at the edges of the transplant. Even transplanted nerves not connected to the trigeminal nerve, the nerve that brings sensation from the face to the brain, recovered sensation.

As Robertson pricked him and observed his responses, she gained insight into Andy's character. She discovered in him a positive and friendly personality. "Anything we asked him to do, he would do," she said. Whether doctors wanted him to meet colleagues in groups or individually, he would roll with it. She found him gracious and easygoing.

This even-tempered personality served Andy well during a recovery that has often vexed other face transplant patients. Recovery from face transplant is significantly different from recovery from solid organ transplant. People who receive solid organ transplants often have serious illnesses, such as kidney or liver disease, that are not outwardly visible to others. For most, their goal is survival, and if the solid organ transplant works, that goal is achieved. In addition, many solid organ recipients experience instantly improved health after the transplant.

Face transplant patients follow a different path. Their health problems before surgery—mainly facial dysfunction and disfigurement—have been obvious to others and required adjustments in their lives, but otherwise most of these patients have been healthy and able-bodied. They do not struggle to stay alive. Their goals focus on improving their facial function and appearance. But the face transplant makes them temporarily dependent on others during their recovery, and their benefits arrive only gradually as nerves regenerate and tissues heal. They must relearn how to function. The adaptations demanded of face transplant patients are different at the sixth month after surgery than at the one-year mark, and there are new challenges after two and three years. Meanwhile, the risks and life changes brought by immunosuppression never go away. It is an ordeal that Andy passed through successfully because of his optimistic personality along with his healthy constitution.

Soon Andy was eating soft foods, dressing himself, and showering without help. He felt no craving for alcohol and remained committed to sobriety. He was not exactly committed to following the hospital's dietary regimen, though. He enjoyed a smuggled slice of pizza earlier than some of his caregivers would have approved. But it sent him into ecstasy. One evening the hospital kitchen mistakenly fulfilled his request for a steak. Andy gobbled it down. Making one of his daily evening visits, Mardini saw evidence of the meal. "What are you eating?" he asked. "Is that steak?" Andy confessed that it was. "Please don't do that," Mardini said. He feared that Andy's jawbone had not yet healed enough to attack such a meal. Andy did not repeat his culinary delinquency.

For much of this time, Reed had justified his long stay in Rochester by saying he was retired and wanted to use his time at one of the world's top medical centers to get his teeth cared for. He indeed did that—getting all his teeth pulled and then being fitted for dentures—and appeared in Andy's hospital room the day after his dental appointment despite his pain. Andy told him to go back to his rented room to take it easy, just this one day.

Looking for an outing, Andy and Reed decided to check out a hobby store in Rochester, as they both enjoyed model cars. Reed was still wincing from his recent tooth extractions, and Andy was just starting to figure out how to speak clearly. When they asked the salesclerk about radio-controlled cars, they took turns stumbling over their requests. "The guy said, 'I don't know what you're talking about,'" Andy recalled. Neither he nor Reed enjoyed success in communicating that day.

Andy knew there was more than tooth care behind Reed's long sojourn in Rochester. "Maybe deep down, it was a way for him to make up for anything he did wrong" years earlier, Andy speculated. He welcomed his dad's visits, although he was not sure what Reed did to keep himself occupied when he was not in the hospital room.

Twice daily, Reed made the thirty-five-minute, one-mile round-trip walk between Charter House, a senior living community owned and operated by Mayo Clinic, and the hospital. As Andy's likely caregiver, he had to master the details of Andy's post-hospital care. During Andy's initial months of recovery, few others close to him had been able to visit. Andy's bond with his father deepened. Their time together in Rochester helped establish a stronger relationship that continued upon Andy's return to Wyoming, where father and son would fish together countless times and regain comfort with each other.

At the end of three months, Reed could no longer remain in Rochester. He had his home to care for, and he had not seen his dog in all that time. "[Andy] was doing well," Reed recalled. "He was in good shape." Andy thought Reed had fulfilled his fatherly duty, and did not feel bad when Reed had to leave.

In his dad's absence, Andy filled his time by playing cribbage with nurses, watching TV, and walking the halls of the hospital. On his first visit to the facility's gym, his physical weakness astonished him. "I couldn't even do a triceps dip," he said. His preoperative 175-pound frame, built by daily trips to a gym in Wyoming, had grown scrawny.

As expected, when Salinas examined Andy's new teeth soon after the transplant, he found extensive cavities, gum disease, and misaligned teeth. As Salinas began correcting these problems, he realized the dental guidelines on treating patients after face transplant were scant. His work on Andy would be pioneering. It was just the challenge for Salinas, who loved to investigate how things worked and who, as a kid, had always been playing with models and clocks and loved science and art. He filled the cavities and removed the tartar from the teeth. "The majority of these teeth were miraculously restorable," he said. In an unanticipated benefit, Salinas could treat Andy's teeth and gums without Novocaine or other anesthetics because the patient still had no sensation in his mouth. Andy received several sessions of restorative dentistry.

Consulting with Mardini and others on the team, Salinas believed fitting Andy with metal braces or other hardware would be unwise because of the risk of irritation to the mouth tissues.

Orthodontist John Volz began working with Andy to consider other ways to straighten his teeth. Andy's medical team had two big concerns. First, would the transplanted blood network supplying his upper and lower jaws tolerate that much structural movement? And second, would the process of adjusting the position of Andy's teeth trigger inflammation and rejection? After consulting with Mardini and Amer, Volz decided to straighten Andy's teeth using clear plastic aligners. Volz discovered that transplanted teeth moved and adjusted a little slower than he expected, but they did eventually align. The work of Volz and Salinas on Andy's teeth was novel for a face transplant patient, and it broke new ground in the field of face transplantation.

Andy's recovery was progressing, but did he look "normal" yet? A significant moment arrived for Andy several months after the transplant. Waiting in line at a grocery store in Rochester, he encountered a man who was studying his face. "Did you get in a car wreck?" the stranger asked. To this unsolicited query, Andy replied, "No, man, it's a little bigger than that." Andy felt elated because it never occurred to the questioner that Andy's face was not the face he was born with. This new kind of interaction and functioning was exactly the type of success Mardini wanted for his patient. He hoped people would talk with Andy, serve him in restaurants and shops, or see him on the street and not have a hint of the medical miracle he represented.

Another important encounter buoyed Andy's spirits. He was riding in a hospital elevator when a fellow passenger, a little boy, looked up at him. In suspense, Andy waited for the boy's reaction. His earlier encounters with children, before the face transplant, had been painful for him. He had often met with looks of fear and hurtful comments. This time, the child turned back to the adult accompanying him without appearing curious, distressed, or frightened—and with no words spoken. "I knew then that the surgery was a success," Andy later told a reporter.

Sometimes Andy's Mayo care team resisted outside excursions. They did not want people staring at him in public. "I'm like, 'Come on, man, you guys are killing me,'" Andy said. "I didn't want to be cooped up all the time, and nobody's going to know anything." He got his hair cut and left the hospital for excursions more and more. Before the face transplant, he had tried to be invisible when in public. "I wouldn't even ask for help," he remembered. He had avoided cities and crowds, but "now I could handle it." He stopped worrying about stares. "Now everybody stares at me normal." His urge to spend time in the outdoors grew powerful. As the cold winter months came on in late 2016, he went ice fishing with his friends Cody and Jeff. One day Andy visited Cody's farm and the goats raised there.

Before Andy's return to Wyoming, Mardini wanted him to have substantial innervation in his face—a recovery of movement and feeling in the transplanted tissue. Lack of innervation to facial muscles caused an unanimated appearance—what Elizabeth Bradley called a "hound dog look"—as evidenced in the early public appearances of some previous face transplant patients.

Mardini and Bradley also wanted to address other concerns before Andy's departure. Once Andy's facial swelling had lessened after the transplant, he was left with excess skin under his eyes, as well as another condition called telecanthus: a wide bridge of skin between the inside corners of the eyes. That month, Mardini and Bradley fixed the telecanthus, improved Andy's tear drainage system, put together the nerves that provided sensation to the midface, and placed custom implants for his lower eye sockets. Some of these improvements had originally been planned for the face transplant surgery, but Mardini and Bradley had postponed them to keep swelling from compressing Andy's eyeballs and compromising his vision. In addition, Andy underwent an operation to align his left eye to prevent double vision.

Bradley's connection to Andy was strong. She, along with Mardini, Amer, and photographer Eric Sheahan, were with Andy on the first Christmas after the transplant. Christmas was often a dark time of the year for Andy, coinciding with the anniversary of his suicide attempt ten years earlier. Yet Andy inspired others around him. "There's just a love for Andy that goes above what you have for the average patient," Bradley observed. John Noseworthy, Mayo's CEO at the time, recalled going to Andy's room for a visit in November 2016. Noseworthy called the meeting "one of the most emotionally powerful moments of my professional life." Andy astonished him. "His persona, his humanity, was being reflected by a transplanted face," said Noseworthy, who knew of Andy's reclusive life before the face transplant. Despite Andy's difficulty in doing such things as blinking and speaking clearly, "you could see him blossoming."

By February 2017, eight months following his transplant, Andy's facial muscles had greatly strengthened in physical therapy. Much innervation had returned. Because he now had a nose with openings, he could smell again and breathe freely. He could eat foods that previously had been difficult for him to chew, including steak, pizza, popcorn, and apples.

Marissa Suchyta, although not on Andy's primary care team, had seen him frequently after his transplant to research the return of sensation to his face and give him surveys to measure the quality of his life. She saw his gains in confidence even in the initial months of his recovery. The highlight of her time with Andy came when it was clear to her that his face was truly functional. When he first smiled, she thought about all the tiny little nerves, connected during the transplant, that made this simple expression— one most of us take for granted—possible. "I remember him telling me he was so happy that he could see children without kids being scared" of him, she said. She could see that he was comfortable with himself, and it made her happy to see him unafraid to go out among people.

As time progressed, Andy grew more emotionally comfortable in his recovery. Mayo initially delayed any release of information on his case and cloistered him in the ICU not only to keep the media at a distance but also to give Andy the chance to adjust to his situation at his own pace. Eventually, however, he approved a limited public release of his story. He did not want a lot of media attention. He chose an approach in which Mayo worked with a single outside journalist to start telling his tale. "We chose a reporter who was a features reporter, not a health reporter," communications manager Ginger Plumbo said. "[Andy and the team] wanted this to be an inspirational story about Andy, and yes, it's interesting medically, but that, we felt, was secondary."

The first interview went to Associated Press reporter Sharon Cohen. She and her AP colleagues did the interview with Andy and shot video footage simultaneously. Cohen's print story began appearing in newspapers nationwide in mid-February 2017. Andy and Mayo declined all other interview requests for Andy that came immediately after the article was published—and there were many of them. But Andy's care team did grant interviews of their own, and Mayo offered parts of its photo and video collection to the media. About two thousand media outlets published either the AP story or the resources from Mayo. When Andy was ready to be discharged, he lived independently for a brief period near the hospital in a Mayo-owned residence. He walked all around Rochester. Nobody harassed him or asked what had happened to him. No paparazzi lay in wait.

Changes within Andy were obvious to many people close to him. No longer a quiet person not wanting to be seen, he recovered his natural exuberance and love of company. "I thought he was an introvert," recalled Arendt, "but as I got to know him, I think he's an extrovert. He seemed very social to me. Anybody that met him just seemed to fall in love with him. He [has] a witty sense of humor. It was fun seeing him pushing the envelope about wanting to get out of the [hospital] room, to interact and be social with others." In the process, Andy acquired a new close circle. "He calls us his Mayo family," Lori Schacht said.

Eight months after his face transplant, Andy attended a Minnesota Wild hockey game at Xcel Energy Center in St. Paul. As he sat in the arena, eating popcorn with thousands of other fans around him, he looked around at the crowd. No one gawked at him; nobody leaned over to whisper a comment to a companion. Everybody was focused on the game, and Andy was relieved to do that, too. He felt like another face in the crowd. It was glorious.

"I don't have to live in fear anymore. I can go out and be myself. I'm allowed to be myself again," said Andy, who had lived for ten years as a recluse out of necessity, out of self-protection. Still, Andy did not believe that he deserved a face transplant more than others with similar needs. "There are hundreds and probably thousands of people that deserve it more," he said. He acknowledges his luck to be chosen for the surgery and the hard work he put in to prepare for it, but Andy does not take his new face for granted. The second chance he received is a treasure to him.

The cost of Andy's face transplant evaluations and surgery was high. The months of postoperative care added significantly to the bill. Andy's employer-provided health insurance would not cover the costs, as the insurer—like many others—considered the treatment investigative and not part of the normal standard of care, despite Mardini's and Amer's communications to the contrary and Mardini's meeting with the CEO of the insurer. Instead, the transplant was made possible by Mayo Clinic's charity care.

Just before Andy's departure from Mayo, the staff threw a surprise birthday party for him. People who were on duty came in their uniforms, and those off duty showed up in their street clothes. Everyone ate cake and took uncountable photos. "I was genuinely shocked," Andy said. "I did not expect that." He had enjoyed his time at Mayo. "I actually didn't want to leave," he said.

When Andy at last left the hospital for Wyoming in February 2017, he took with him a multitude of memories from his time at Mayo. One image stood out from his early weeks of recovery, when he was often in a medicated fog. He frequently hallucinated, believing that a spy occupied his room and that a camera on the wall was recording his every move. Even while in a chair, he would doze off and wake up repeatedly. "I don't remember a whole lot from those first days, but I remember one time I sat in the chair, and I woke up," he said. A nurse, Kim, stood before him, ready to brush his teeth. "Who is this girl? Wow," he thought. He feared looking at her directly, he thought she was so beautiful.

Kim, who grew up on a sixty-head dairy farm in Cannon Falls, Minnesota, an hour's drive from Rochester, had earned her nursing degree from Winona State University. After working in an assisted living facility, she joined Mayo Clinic. Though she had never worked in the ICU before Andy's arrival, she responded to a request from a nursing administrator for additional plastic surgery nurses to support the ICU team for Andy's case. Kim was warned, "You can't talk about this assignment." She agreed, unaware of the identity of her future patient. When she walked into his ICU room on her first shift and saw him lying unconscious on his bed, she was moved by his helplessness and the long recovery that lay ahead for him.

Her heart took over, "which can be good and bad in certain situations," she said. "I think it makes me caring and compassionate. And patients feel that." With Andy, it was no different. "I saw his strength and felt empathy for what he had been through for the past ten years and hope for him, for his future." During more relaxed shifts, as Andy recovered, she began to see him as more of a person, even though he could not yet speak.

"When you're working closely for so long, you start to open up," Kim said. She found herself talking with Andy about her life. She felt drawn to Andy but pushed her thoughts of him away. Romance—especially with a patient—was not on her mind. Andy left the ICU in mid-July 2016, and Kim did not see him again until the week he left the hospital. A question mark accompanied her thoughts of Andy.

At last—looking something like Matt Damon, as some of his friends thought—Andy went home to Wyoming and his new life.

# Chapter 11

# Liberation

———

Now living in Cheyenne, Wyoming, Andy felt liberated. When he went into restaurants he could order steak, pizza, and other foods—all formerly impossible for him to consider eating with his old, reconstructed face. Other diners did not stare at him with curious or troubled expressions. In his dreams, he continued to see himself with his new face—a remarkably fast incorporation of his changed physical appearance into his sense of personal identity. "It's part of me," he said. "It's my face." The world's thirty-ninth face transplant patient (the twelfth in the United States) at last had accomplished his goal of a functional face that allowed him to live with the anonymity he craved.

Andy rented a little basement apartment and resumed lifting weights at a local gym. His weight had dropped thirty pounds and he needed to recover his strength after so long in the hospital. The immunosuppressive medications caused him to tire easily, but he kept up his workouts.

Meanwhile, his social life quickly flourished. In the past, he'd often avoided people, finding it easier to hide than to explain his appearance or discuss what he'd been through. No more. He started diving into things he had missed for years: freely socializing, dancing, eating out, going to concerts. He even went back to camping, something he had stopped because his prosthetic nose kept going missing in the woods.

Now he was catching up on all the things he had shied away from due to unwanted attention. With his old face, just being in public had grown too difficult. He had become averse to other people. But things had changed. "There's not one part of me that still thinks I'm not normal," he said. The once reclusive Andy was now blossoming. Simple accomplishments—smiling, kissing— delighted him. Gradually, his sense of taste returned, and his sense of smell was not far behind.

"There's no part of me that's uncomfortable anymore," he said. "There's no situation that I don't want to be in anymore." Andy's family saw the change in his mood and approach to life. "We don't have to worry about you anymore," his brother, Ronald, told him. Everyone could recognize the difference between what he looked like before and after the transplant, but it was equally apparent how much Andy's personality had freed itself from its old restraints. After the facial reconstruction that followed his suicide attempt, "I had to become an asshole to survive"—to develop a tough shell—"because people were picking on me and making fun of me," Andy said. "I had to be mean." With his new face, Andy became open, gregarious, and happy to engage with others. "It turns out Andy is not as much of an introvert as we thought," Mardini told a reporter.

Andy often traveled from Cheyenne to visit Ronald's family in Newcastle, and to celebrate holidays there, playing with his five-year-old niece, Valerie, riding in a side-by-side all-terrain vehicle with his dad, and just hanging out. Andy always found time to attend his nephew Luke's wrestling matches and baseball games. And he kept up with his older sister, Rhiannon, who lived in West Virginia, during frequent phone conversations. About his family, Andy said proudly: "They know that I'm going to be fine."

Andy believed that all the hard work that had gone into the planning and performance of the face transplant and his recovery had realized his best hopes. "I've had three different faces, been three different people," he said. He would always have to combat depression, for which he took medication, but he believed he had come a long way from 2006.

Andy's daily routine now included new habits. He practiced gently massaging his face in patterns his physical therapists had suggested, to stimulate his still-connecting nerves. As his speech therapist urged, while showering or working around the house, he recited out loud the letters of the alphabet, to improve his speech. He worked on actively moving his lower jaw when he talked, which made his speech clearer. To combat his left eye's synkinesis—the movement of the eye upward when he blinked—he practiced closing his eyelid slowly and concentrating on preventing the eye from moving when the lid opened.

He divided his waking hours by calculating when he had to take his immunosuppressants and other medications. He would think, "OK, so it's five o'clock. Let's do the math. When should I take my 750 milligrams of [immunosuppressant] mycophenolate? How many am I allowed to take between now and nine o'clock? I parcel out the meds so I have something in my system and I'm not overdoing it. Because overdosing could damage my kidneys."

He carried his pills in his pocket and set alarms on his phone reminding him of when to take the medicine. His tactics worked most of the time. "You're not going to get your meds in all the time perfectly," he said, "but as long as you can stay close to your time and not miss doses, that's the biggest thing." During the first four years after Andy's return home, he said he missed only two doses.

Andy also had to be careful with his diet. Eating certain citrus fruits—such as grapefruit, some kinds of oranges, and large amounts of clementines—could interfere with the way his body metabolized his medications, leading to potentially dangerous levels in his body. Fortunately, Andy was not that fond of clementines.

He also had to take an antifungal drug that demanded both a food chaser and a cola chaser to increase its absorption. Sushi was off-limits because of its potential to introduce infectious agents to his immunosuppressed system. Often, however, he ignored the restriction on sushi. "I eat it all the time," Andy confessed. "I love it." He became a fanatical user of hand sanitizer, which, he hoped, had the effect of counteracting any pathogens coming from the sushi. It would not have that effect, but Andy never experienced any problems from the raw fish.

Andy had used much of his recovery time in Rochester to study for his electrician's licensing exam. Now back in Cheyenne, he returned to work for All Electric as a third-year electrician apprentice, working for the area's oil and gas developers. Later he won a promotion to lead electrician. He then rose to become a licensed journeyman electrician. Everywhere he worked, he received support. A coworker, Mike, became a roommate and close friend Andy could lean on. Andy lost his old fear of explaining himself on the job and his worry about how others would see him.

Andy also maintained a side business as a welder, creating sheet metal panel boards for his employer to use in the oil fields. He built them in a one-car garage in his apartment complex. Some of the panels he wrangled weighed five hundred pounds. There were weeks he worked more than seventy hours in his day job while welding panel boards at night and on the weekend. His goal was to save up enough money to buy a utility all-terrain vehicle.

Andy's relationship with Kim, the nurse at Mayo with whom he had become smitten, had remained "professional," he said, during his ICU stay. After he left the hospital, Kim still thought of him. She could picture hanging out with him along with her friends. They started talking on the phone, as friends, a couple of months after his discharge. Although they were 850 miles apart, Kim soon realized she was falling in love with him.

"I want to come out," she told him in one call. He welcomed the idea of a visit from her and helped her plan the details of her trip. But he remained unconvinced that Kim was truly serious about her visit. Kim was serious, though, and she saw her forthcoming visit as a defining event. "I'm either going to come back knowing that I'll never have feelings for this guy more than as a friend," she said, "or I'm going to come back feeling head-over-heels for him."

Arriving in Cheyenne, she texted him saying she was standing outside his apartment, and where was *he?* Andy, still not quite sure she was really coming, had gone to work. Disbelieving, he asked her to send him a photo of herself outside the residence. "She was there," he said. She had flown to Denver, rented a car, and driven to Cheyenne, just as they had planned. He gave her the passcode to his front door. "The next thing I know, I come home from work and she's in my living room." He was shocked and happy—"it was way sweet," he said—because he had not had a romantic involvement with anyone since before his initial injury in 2006.

On the spur of the moment, they decided to make a getaway to Estes Park, Colorado, for the weekend. They bonded on the trip, and Kim ate mussels for the first time. She liked trying new foods— one of many traits she shared with Andy.

When she and Andy became seriously involved in August 2017, they traded visits with each other and kept things going long distance for two years. Andy's deepening self-esteem and confidence impressed Kim. She appreciated how he could walk up to anyone and start a conversation. It hurt her to imagine all the years in which he had isolated himself. "He bloomed completely out of his shell, and thank God he was given an opportunity to do that," she said.

"She saw the will I had to live through all that I've lived through while still being happy and fun," Andy said. "I was still myself." Andy believed they were alike in important ways. Besides eating adventurously, they both liked fishing, hunting, camping, travel, and swimming. They adored kids; Kim saw the love that passed between Andy and his niece and nephew, Ronald's children.

She also was witness to Andy's fond relationship with Mardini, which she called "adorable." "He cares so much about Andy, and it's reflected in their phone calls," she said. Patient and doctor kept in touch through video calls in which Andy offered tips on fishing, among their other topics of conversation unrelated to medicine. "All my children love to fish, but I don't really know how to fish," Mardini said, "so I call him to ask for advice." Kim considered their patient-doctor friendship a treasure: "They sometimes don't talk for months at a time, but when they do, they just pick up right where they left off," she said.

Kim moved to Wyoming to be with Andy in 2019. Their relationship grew deeper in each other's constant presence: they planned date nights, had dinners out, and hung out. "We were meant to be together," Andy said. They married on May 30, 2020, in a ceremony at Terry Peak, in Deadwood, South Dakota—roughly the midpoint between the places where they grew up. Andy had wished to get married on the actual mountaintop, but they settled for exchanging vows in a nearby resort at a lower altitude in the Black Hills. COVID-19 precautions prevented many of Andy's Mayo care team members and other friends from attending, although photographer Eric Sheahan was there to capture images. Mardini became emotional when he later saw the photos, which included a portrait of the newlyweds in front of a waterfall. Mardini could not stop looking at Andy's happy facial expressions, which would have been impossible for Andy before the transplant.

The wedding fulfilled one of Andy's goals for his face transplant. "One of the main reasons why I did it was to get a wife, have kids, and have my own family one day," he said. That part was not far off. Andy and Kim soon announced that Kim was pregnant. They chose not to find out the baby's sex in advance, so Andy chose a boy's name and Kim selected a girl's. The child, a boy, was born in October 2020.

Andy felt happy to once again live close to his brother, Ronald. Together they had been through a rough childhood that had given them a strong bond. Their mother's death had drawn them together even more closely. They were confident in their support for each other, but not big on conversation. They simply accepted each other, helped each other, and remained locked in as family members. Kim observed they had "a brotherhood that will never go away."

Andy returned to Rochester many times for follow-up procedures and treatment. Salinas marveled at how well Andy maintained his dental hygiene, given the numbness he continued to experience in parts of his mouth. Even so, one of his teeth was not salvageable and had to be replaced by a dental implant. In his consultations with orthodontist Volz, Andy continued to be fitted with dental aligners, worn during waking hours, to improve the alignment of his teeth. Andy's mouth cavity was loaded with invisible but permanent hardware—screws, bolts, clips—from the transplant surgery, but it was all underneath the surface. Andy's dental X-rays were striking as a result, but they did not faze the orthodontist, who had plenty of experience working with facial reconstruction patients.

Andy's eyes also needed attention. At one point, he began to experience constant tearing, which interfered with the fine detail of his work as an electrician and handicapped his hunting in the winter chill of Wyoming's outdoors. In a follow-up surgery, Mardini and Bradley found a mass of scar tissue below his eyes around the tear duct network that drained fluid from his eyes to his nose. The connection between Rudy's tissue and Andy's tissue had become scarred and needed repair. Bradley and Mardini reconstructed the area using a microscope and sutures as thin as a human hair. Andy's tearing improved after that, despite needing a few follow-ups. He had 20/20 vision in his right eye and less acuity in his left eye, but did not need eyeglasses, and could drive noncommercial vehicles safely.

A minor immunological reaction prompted another visit to Mayo. After wearing a harness while working on an oil field tower, Andy noticed small red bumps on the sentinel flap transplanted into his groin area. The rubbing and pressure from the harness had created inflammation, which triggered a rejection episode on the groin flap, but not on the face. Andy consulted with Amer, who suggested keeping an eye on it for a few days. When the skin of the signal flap did not improve, Andy went back to Rochester, where he underwent a biopsy that confirmed a rejection. He received high-dose steroids, which resolved the episode.

Andy also returned to Mayo for twice-yearly checkups that lasted two or three days. He initially disliked these visits because he was not sick, the exams fatigued him, and the scrutiny he received seemed a waste of time. Then he realized these visits were an opportunity to see his friends at Mayo, not to mention help medical science. "I know all these guys like family. They're family to me," he said. His care team shared that feeling. "Andy says we changed his life, but he changed ours," said Mardini. "We appreciate the small things that make a difference." With each visit, Andy suffered less of the dreaded poking and prodding. Blood draws were always to be expected, but Andy bargained with Amer to receive blood draws less frequently as long as his drug regimen did not change. Sometimes Andy had skin biopsies done. He met with psychiatrist Jowsey-Gregoire, who in talking with Andy used the simile that life is like a sawblade, constantly rising and falling.

Andy would have his ups and downs in a never-ending cycle, and his task was to expect, plan for, and handle the low points.

Andy grew to look forward to his Mayo visits. "Actually, it's fun," he said. He liked to gather with groups of his caregivers to see friendly faces and shake hands. Some of his favorite people there were starting to retire. It helped that Andy drove to and from Minnesota with his dog Blue, a springerdoodle. All along the way, in stops for food and fuel, people loved Blue, even though the dog was "a scaredy cat," according to Andy.

An unusual meeting brought Andy one of the most unforgettable memories of his face transplant experience. Near the time of Andy's hospital discharge in the fall of 2016, Lilly Ross, the widow of Andy's face donor, Rudy Ross, had written a set of letters to all the recipients of Rudy's organs. Lilly was nineteen years old and eight months pregnant when Rudy (or "Rude," as she sometimes called him) died. "I am filled with great joy knowing that he was able to give a little of himself to ensure a better quality of life for someone else," Andy read in the letter he received. Lilly told of Rudy's love of hunting, trapping, and spending time with Grit, his dog. With Andy's OK, LifeSource gave Lilly photos showing Andy before and after his transplant. In one photo, Lilly noticed a familiar feature on Andy's healing face: a bare spot on the chin in the middle of the beard—a patch of skin Rudy's face also possessed. But this was the only real similarity between the faces of the two men after the transplant. (A 2018 study published in a medical journal concluded that few face transplant recipients resemble their donors because of differences in facial bone structure and other factors.)

Andy received photos of Rudy and his family as well, including a picture of Lilly and Rudy's infant son. Andy noticed how Rudy's face matched Andy's pre-injury face. In the photos of Rudy, it was startling how close the skin tone, hair color, and facial features of the two men had been. "We could be brothers and hang out," Andy said. "Dead serious." He later saw a photo of Rudy posing with a shotgun in hand. "This guy could be my twin, honestly. He has the same posture, same everything."

Andy also learned for the first time that Rudy had taken his own life, knowledge that gave extra meaning to the photos. Andy had hoped that his donor's face would come to him in another way, such as after a car accident. Mardini and Jowsey-Gregoire gave Andy the information gently, yet it stunned Andy into a few minutes of silence. "He looked at me in deep thought, trying to process what he had heard," Mardini said. "He then changed completely." Andy said the knowledge of Rudy's suicide made his organ donations even more significant and gave Andy a stronger connection with Rudy's family. "I know what they're going through even more, because I know what my family went through," Andy said.

He grieved with Lilly. "He changed a lot of lives. I'm glad I'm one," Andy said. He let Lilly know he hoped he would meet her someday. He mentioned that he believed Rudy, in some sense, would continue doing the hunting and fishing he loved, through Andy. He did not know what had made Rudy take his own life. Both men had been twenty-one when they shot themselves.

Lilly and Andy did meet, in October 2017, a year and four months after the transplant. The visit was arranged by LifeSource and Mayo in the wood-paneled Plummer Library on the Mayo campus. Lilly brought along her toddler, Leonard, because she wanted him to witness (and later understand) how much Rudy's organ donations had helped other people.

Both Andy and Lilly were nervous during the meeting. "I am terrified, but I am excited," Lilly said while she waited for Andy to appear. Andy, although he does not normally sweat excessively, noticed that his armpits were drenched. He had slept poorly the night before, and he felt tense. He thought his face looked drained of color. He entered the library and they hugged. Her eyes were wet, and the tension eased.

"You look really good," Lilly said.

"Thank you so much," Andy replied. He added, "I wanted to show you that your gift will not be wasted."

Everybody in the room was crying. Other than Rudy's distinctive beard gap, she said, she saw only Andy. Together they looked at photos of her family, and Andy held Leonard in his arms. Andy shared the gains he was making in speaking and eating, and that he sometimes went out dancing.

Lilly made one request of Andy: to touch his face. Andy consented and closed his eyes as Lilly's hand approached. "It feels really good," she said. Among the people watching, Mayo communications manager Ginger Plumbo found the moment touching and surreal. "I am extremely proud of Rude that he was able to help numerous people, with the heart, the liver, the lungs, the kidneys, the pancreas," Lilly said later, not to mention the miraculous gift of a face.

After everyone left the library, Andy and Lilly had lunch together, along with Lilly's mother and sister, as well as Leonard, away from the cameras. They talked and got to know each other. "She's just the strongest girl I know," Andy said. They took a group picture in the restaurant, and while Andy walked with them to their car, Lilly said, "Hey, I've got something for you." She reached into the car and handed Andy a bag of Rudy's cremated remains. "I want you to spread these in Wyoming because I want him to do the things you do and be at the places you've been," Lilly said. Inexpressibly honored, Andy kept the ashes in his sock drawer for a long time until he found the perfect time and place to spread them. "There's a place where I used to hunt, and it's my favorite place in the whole world," he said. The spot is on the top of a mountain, overlooking fields. "It's so beautiful, and that's the first place that hit my mind."

The publicity surrounding Andy's meeting with Lilly, the result of rolling video and clicking cameras, was part of Mayo's ongoing overall effort to manage media interest in Andy. Journalists reporting on the meeting depended on the institution for access, using photos and video footage provided by Mayo.

Mayo had committed to fielding the media inquiries that came in over the long term. On Andy's behalf, "we have declined a ton of requests for interviews with him, without even bothering him about it," said Ginger Plumbo. The strategy worked. After leaving the hospital, Andy was not bombarded with media requests, and no reporter tried to call his cellphone to snag an interview. Instead, Mayo periodically released updates on his progress, which appeared thousands of times in the media.

In 2020, the COVID-19 pandemic engulfed the world. Andy's immunosuppression placed him at particular risk of infection. He successfully avoided the virus and its variants by masking and through his devotion to hand sanitizer. Meanwhile, the price of oil dropped, and oil-related employment crashed throughout the mountain states and the Upper Midwest. People in Andy's line of work had their hours cut or eliminated. "I said I'm done with it," Andy observed. "I'm not going to work in the oil field anymore."

Andy saw the economic downturn as a hidden gift—a chance for him and Kim to take a new direction. They talked about moving to Minnesota. Andy would miss his family and friends in Wyoming, but he liked the idea of being closer to Kim's family. In a lucky moment, Andy received a job offer in Minnesota that used his skills well, and soon after, Kim took an opportunity to return to her nursing job at Mayo Clinic. Together, they relocated to southern Minnesota. Andy loves going back to Wyoming to visit everybody he knows there. But he insists it was a smart decision to branch out on his own.

# Chapter 12

# Fear Is Gone

———

Andy had always felt nervous about speaking in public. For a long time after his face transplant, he was reluctant to even consider the prospect of talking before an audience. But it was through a series of speaking engagements that Andy learned how to reflect on his life with others and grow more comfortable appearing before large groups.

His very first speaking engagement had been for LifeSource, before a group of two hundred transplant physicians and administrators. It was less than a year after his transplant. "I'd never in my life been in front of two hundred people, so that one was nerve-racking," he says. "I remember when I stepped off the stage, I just started shaking. I was so nervous, so relieved it was over."

On another occasion, he addressed the Mayo board of trustees. The trustees could not believe what they were hearing. Many were in tears. "He held the audience breathless for twenty minutes or a half hour," former Mayo CEO John Noseworthy said.

In September 2019, he agreed to appear onstage at a conference that attracted four hundred healthcare and technology leaders to the Civic Center in Rochester. Transform 2019, as the conference was called, was a two-day investigation of innovative changes in the delivery and practice of healthcare. Mardini and Jowsey-Gregoire joined Andy before an audience to discuss the many novel aspects of his face transplant and Andy's recovery from it.

The physicians gave their perspectives on preparing for Andy's surgery, how it went, and the significance of the face transplant in medical practice. Andy then described his experience and how his new face had affected his life. "When I first saw it," he told the Transform attendees, "I'll never forget just looking in that mirror. Just wow. That's all I could say, was 'wow.'" He told the crowd about his mental state before he shot himself in 2006, how he kept himself apart from his friends and family for months. How he bottled up his emotions and did not seek psychiatric help. And how he allowed his feelings to explode out and spark a crisis that nearly claimed his life. He told them how he had regretted his suicide attempt the instant he pulled the trigger.

Not many people survive a suicide attempt in such a manner. Andy overcame his anxiety over public speaking to urge others to seek help instead of contemplating suicide. By talking about his perilous journey, Andy was convinced, he could help other struggling people. "If you are feeling these thoughts and feelings, you just need to get it out there and you need to talk to someone," he told the audience. He felt strongly that encouraging even a single person to seek help would be worthwhile.

At the same time, Andy did not present himself as an all-knowing guru. He admitted on the stage that he was still uncertain about his purpose in life, although he thought that urging people to choose hope and life over death might be part of it. "I was nervous about this today," he confessed to the audience. "If I could tell something to anyone who is feeling the way that I felt, it's that you have to find these feelings and identify them and face them for what they are. If you are feeling these thoughts, you have to talk to someone, and it can be anyone." After the Transform presentation, Andy received a standing ovation.

In appearances with Mardini, Andy preferred their presentation to seem like an informal discussion. They would talk back and forth almost as if there was no audience. The plastic surgeon always emphasized that as the patient, Andy was the one people should hear from about his medical treatment. He had the experience and perspective that hardly anyone else on earth possessed. As time went by, Andy's speaking anxieties diminished.

Away from audiences, Andy admits it was difficult to tell people considering suicide to talk about their feelings with others, knowing he had so fatefully ignored such advice. "I knew that I should just talk to somebody," he says. He wonders whether his public speaking truly could have the effect of steering desperate people in a better direction. "They have to have that awakening themselves," he says.

Still, he hopes he might be the person who changes the mind of someone in crisis. Over time Andy has shifted his public talks from a recounting of his experiences as a face transplant patient to something with a pay-it-forward message. He offers inspiration and hope to other people in despair. He raises awareness of the importance of mental health, ways to deal with depression, and how to avoid suicide. That message is needed. Suicide is the second-leading cause of death for Americans between twenty and twenty-four years old, the age range that included Andy when he shot himself. "When you decide you want to commit suicide," Andy says, "you feel like the world is better off without you. That's just the way you feel. You feel like there's nothing you could do to contribute to society, you're just worthless. That's how I felt." Looking back, he now recognizes all the people who were willing to help and support him—a help network he did not understand he had when he was twenty-one.

Speaking to a Department of Defense healthcare group for veterans, he urged the attendees to make face transplants available to military patients. Although facially wounded patients are usually not in immediate danger of dying, Andy made clear he considers a face transplant a lifesaving procedure. "If I had looked like I did for the rest of my life, I'm not living life to the fullest," he said. "And that was the point."

Sometimes at these events, Andy tells memorable anecdotes. At one meeting of transplant physicians and administrators, he spoke about the relief he felt that children no longer looked at him with obvious fear and anxiety. As someone who loves spending time with children, this change brought him tremendous relief. He also remarked that he was happy to jump on a trampoline without his old prosthetic nose flying off.

Although the story Andy tells his audiences of his injury, reconstruction, and face transplant is nearly unique in human experience, its broad outlines are not uncommon in the world. Anyone at any time could make an impulsive decision—out of anger or frustration, or under the influence of drink or drugs—changing the course of everything afterward. For young people, impulsiveness almost comes naturally. Because the frontal lobes of their brains—brain structures critical in decision-making—are not yet fully developed, people under twenty-five are especially prone to making irrational decisions.

The universal aspect of Andy's talks is what resonates most in the people who hear it. Learning about his experience can help anyone with similar depressed and self-destructive feelings, anyone who has made a mistake with serious consequences. That's a large share of us. We are not perfect or indestructible. Each of us will have a time when our body or mind fails us. When that difficult time comes, we must recognize it, solve the problem it presents, find and accept the support of others, and cultivate our natural resilience. In the process, we may have to make steps into the unknown. It does no good to burden ourselves with guilt. Andy's experience tells us that second chances do come.

After the flurry of speaking engagements that began during his recovery from his face transplant, Andy backed off from public talks. Although he enjoys giving public presentations, he wanted to focus on his own life. Now married, with two children, living in an area different from his native Wyoming, he wanted to get his life organized. Eventually, Andy thinks, he might yet return to public speaking. "I actually wouldn't mind doing it full-time," he says. He feels proud of all he has accomplished in his public outreach, and he suspects there is more he can do.

When they moved to Minnesota, Andy and Kim settled into a farmhouse in Cannon Falls, located on property belonging to Kim's father. Their dog chased cats all day.

Andy started working as an electrician for a residential solar panel company, installing panels around the Twin Cities. Some of the work is outdoors, and "Dr. Amer would probably not appreciate that," Andy says. He usually works on the ground, installing electrical mounts, while others work on the roofs. He drinks plenty of water, and as far as his transplant team knows, a big sombrero-style hat shades him when the sun blasts.

A huge difference from the past is that he no longer worries about whether he fits in and if his coworkers will accept him. "I can do my job. I can focus," he says. Away from work, "I can think about life and reminisce about old times when I'm driving and listen to the radio and actually enjoy it." He does not feel anxiety over decisions that previously plagued him, such as where he will go to eat or whether people will understand him when he speaks. He no longer worries over what other people think of his appearance. His main concern now is managing all the medications he takes.

Andy and Kim had their first child, Wyatt Lee, in October 2020. "I've never expected that to happen in my whole life," Andy says. Wyatt's arrival inspired Andy—accustomed to working long, hard hours—to cut down on his time on the job. Andy reveled in holding his baby and walking around with him. Before the birth of his son, Andy had been afraid to touch infants. They always seemed to start crying once in his arms. "When Wyatt was born, all of that went away," he says.

Today, Andy wants to be a good father, and he already anticipates working on cars and sharing other experiences with his son. "I want to make sure he understands that if he has any problems, he can come talk to me—I'd be judgment-free," Andy says. There is nothing he would not do for his kid. That first holiday season with Wyatt in 2020—which included the anniversaries of his mother's death and Andy's suicide attempt—passed without Andy feeling depressed about either past event. In previous Decembers, he would frequently break down crying. Now he had his young family to live for.

Kim was responsible for most of the parenting time, but as Wyatt grew, he and his dad developed a routine. On weekends, they watched TV for an hour or so before going outdoors. Even on very cold days, Wyatt tolerated the weather. After spending an hour or so outside, they'd come back in and Andy would put Wyatt down for his nap. At night, Wyatt was supposed to be in bed by seven-thirty. In Andy's care, it was often closer to eight-thirty. The time Andy spent with Wyatt reminded him of his own time with Reed, and how his father's work schedule had given them little time together until Andy was older. "That's one of the reasons why I try to be home as much as possible," Andy says. He and Kim later had a second child, a daughter named Grace Catherine.

Reed now visits Andy and Kim every few months from New-castle. Their relationship is strong, and everyone works hard to keep it so. "It means a lot to me. I talk to him at least every other day, three times a week," Andy says.

Andy feels he made the right choice to move to Minnesota for his health and future and for Kim, but he feels responsible for keeping in touch with his family. An unfortunate legacy he received from his upbringing is poor communication habits, though. "We don't know how to talk," he says of his relationship with his brother, Ronald. "We don't know how to talk about feelings." Andy sees Ronald as a good brother, friend, and father, and Andy wants Ronald to understand he appreciates him. Sometimes Andy tries to break the old patterns by texting Ronald that he loves and misses him.

Andy's close relationship with Mardini persists. They are friends who view and keep in touch with each other as brothers. "And I don't think he does it just for the face," Andy says—it is a genuine connection. In addition to their twice-yearly in-person meetings during Andy's checkups, they frequently talk and text. "Who has that kind of relationship with their doctor?" Andy asks. Mardini's wife, Rawan, observes: "Our kids don't think twice—they run and hug Andy because they know he's Samir's friend. We think of him as family."

Mardini feels especially proud of one aspect of Andy's post-transplant life: "We helped him become normal so that he has his normal problems." Yes, Andy's general health is excellent, and he has remarkable function in his face. He has the same kind of challenges and problems that most people have. That makes him a regular guy, "just like you are, just like I am," Mardini says. It is what Andy long yearned for—to mix in, pursue happiness without attracting attention, find a partner and start a family, and feel average. He now has it, a gigantic achievement that some people don't know how to appreciate even when they possess it.

One other facet of Andy's new life astounds Mardini. "When I see him, I can't believe what he looks like. I look at the movements in his face and the emotions he expresses—they appear so natural and effortless," he says. "I think about the miracle that these are the movements of a face that once belonged to someone else, and that person is no longer with us. But this face is living the life of another person." Scientifically, Andy's face transplant was a remarkable event. "But even more remarkable is that this face is allowing Andy to live a normal life. It's giving him a second chance at life, and I love it that Andy is wholeheartedly grateful and takes nothing for granted," Mardini adds.

∼

In 2021, Andy and Kim purchased their own property about five miles from Kim's father's place. Andy calls it a diamond in the rough. Working on weekends over the course of a year, they tore down an old farmhouse (after salvaging its hardwood floorboards) and a couple of wrecked barns, cleared the ground of junk, and planned for the construction of a new house. They were going to build as much of it as possible by hand, on their own. The new parents at times felt torn; some days they wanted to forget about the house and spend their time cuddling with their children. But they resisted often enough. Their new home would be the place where their children would grow up, with Kim's family close at hand.

Excavation of the land for the new house began in June 2021. Meanwhile, Andy and Kim were buying stone and lumber left over from other building projects at half price. From his employer, Andy got solar roof panels at a discount. He looked forward to spending his free summer hours constructing the house. "I know how to work," he says, although he hired out framing, cement work, drywalling, and some other parts of the construction. "It will be nice to just sit down on our porch one night and say, 'Man, we did it,'" Andy says. "We built the house, we got our life."

Andy wonders what he will tell his children about his past when they grow older. He feels nervous about sitting down with older versions of his kids and explaining everything, from his depression and suicide attempt through the face transplant. Andy knows he will have to do it someday, and he does not want his children to hear about it for the first time from other people. "Are they going to lose respect for their dad, or will they gain respect for their dad?" Andy questions. He hopes that by sharing his story and inspiring others, he can help his children feel proud of him and learn to see the good in people.

Andy continues to see his Mayo care team twice a year to monitor the health of his transplanted tissues and the long-term effects of his immunosuppression therapy. Andy now takes eleven different immunosuppression and other medications each day, all orally. He eats and often rests after taking his medicines—if he skips this part, he can get shaky. He avoids grapefruit and other citrus fruits as well as black licorice because they interfere with the metabolism of his medications. Part of his morning ritual is to use a nasal rinse to keep his nose clear. Andy also has restrictions on certain cold and cough medications; it is hard for him to keep track of which ones are safe, so he avoids all of them. Nonsteroidal anti-inflammatory medications, such as ibuprofen, are discouraged because they may damage his kidneys.

"I take my meds on time, and I am mostly fine," he says. "There will be a couple days a month where no matter what I do, I have to let my stomach rest." He does not believe his intensive regimen limits his life or his enjoyment of it.

Many people at Mayo call Andy's story a tale of heroism, perseverance, and sacrifice, because he put his life on the line to join with his caregivers in betting on the benefits of a face transplant. "The whole tale of a traumatized young man who survives an attempt on his life, lives in isolation, and ultimately commits to [the transplant] and regains his place in society and creates a path forward for other people—it's like a fairy tale," declares Noseworthy, who praises the commitment of hundreds of Mayo staff, working together for Andy's benefit, who did not care who got the credit.

Andy's experience reveals much about Mayo Clinic as well. His great outcome shows how the commitment, talents, and full support of a healthcare institution can change a patient's life. There was goodness in the marriage of science and heart, and it was present for Andy.

Andy continues to marvel at his luck in receiving his transplant surgery when other deserving patients did not. "I don't think people realize what this has done for me, how it has made me. I don't have to live in fear anymore. I can go out and be myself," he says. Sometimes, at rare and wonderful moments, he forgets he ever had a face transplant. But then he remembers, and he thinks about Rudy, his donor, and how much that man and his family lost. This train of thought usually leads Andy to the same conclusion: his own life has changed so much for the better. "I wouldn't ever ask for this much, I never would have taken this much, but it was given to me," he says.

# Epilogue

In February 2024, Mardini's team performed the second face transplant at Mayo Clinic. Derek Pfaff, a 30-year-old from Harbor Beach, Michigan, had attempted to take his own life in 2014. Like Andy, Derek's face was left severely damaged by a gunshot. Despite undergoing 58 reconstructive facial surgeries, he was still unable to eat solid food or speak casually with friends and family. Wearing glasses proved impossible without a nose. A face transplant changed all of that.

Led by Mardini, the procedure was carefully choreographed as before, lasting more than 50 hours and involving at least 80 healthcare professionals. The transplant team replaced part of the forehead and virtually everything below Derek's eyebrows, including the eyelids, jaws, teeth, nose, cheek structure, neck skin, the hard palate, and parts of the soft palate. Methodical stitching of muscle to muscle, nerve to nerve, allows Derek to now express a range of emotions on his face.

~

Complex as they are, face transplants will continue, but not for large numbers of patients. "It is for a very select group of individuals who would benefit from the procedure as it stands right now, and who understand the trade-offs [the risks of immunosuppression medication] and can accept those trade-offs for the improved function," Hatem Amer says. Function, Amer still believes, should be the main goal, not aesthetics. Although face transplant is not a death-preventing surgery, that does not mean patients who receive it are healthy in all respects before their operations. Nearly all keep themselves separate from society. Like Andy, they live in isolation because of their disfigurement. And often they are not eating or breathing well, because of the damage caused to their face by injury or illness. These patients need treatment, and face transplant remains an option.

Since the first face transplant in 2006, the procedure has evolved from a curiosity with uncertain outcomes to an effective treatment for patients who are willing to undergo the rigid pharmacological regimen and who can avoid excessive sun exposure, smoking, and other damaging environmental factors. In most cases, the transplants have improved patients' appearance and functionality—and their lives.

Until recently, there have been only two possible outcomes from face transplant surgery: success or, for a few patients, death from tissue rejection and other causes. Even success can eventually take a turn, however. Connie Culp, whose face transplant at the Cleveland Clinic in 2008 made her the first such patient in the United States, died in 2020. News reports said she died from an infection. Her death sparked critical evaluation among people working in face transplant surgery. "Every death that occurs affects the whole field because it is still so new," Mardini says. "We have the responsibility to do everything possible to make it a success not just for the patient, but for the field."

Patients face fewer risks of tissue rejection when their immune systems are not already sensitized to antigens, or foreign substances, in the donor's system. Sensitization creates a risky situation, which is why finding a good match between donor and recipient is so important. After transplant, people who take their immunosuppressive medications on schedule are more likely to do well. In addition, developing healthy habits, such as eating nutritious foods and exercising, gives patients an edge, Mardini believes.

It is terrible when actual tissue rejection occurs. "The body starts fighting the face," Mardini says, "or the face starts fighting the body." The tissues become irreparably damaged as a result. Recent second transplants on the same patient (repeat transplants), however, enlarge the field of possible outcomes by allowing for a repeat procedure. In January 2018, forty-three-year-old Jérôme Hamon, who had neurofibromatosis type 1, a disease that can cause disfiguring and debilitating skin tumors, became the first person to receive a second face transplant after his first transplanted tissue showed signs of severe rejection. French surgeon Laurent Lantieri performed the repeat procedure eight years after the first. Hamon died in 2024.

To avoid rejection and other unwanted outcomes, Mardini has developed a set of criteria for the selection of patients and for the qualities needed in face transplant teams. Patients, he believes, should be fully informed in their transplant decision, in good medical condition, willing to take on the responsibilities of lifelong immunosuppression, psychologically resilient with a strong support network, and willing to accept the risks of transplant surgery. Most important, patients must be courageous. At the same time, face transplant teams must be willing to meet the surgical and anatomic challenges of the procedure, committed to teamwork, and willing to accompany the patient on an extensive and arduous journey.

As for the future treatment of patients like Andy, improvements in immunosuppressive medications could make them less risky and burdensome, and patients' post-transplant lives easier.

Transplantable tissue grown in laboratories from the patient's own stem cells could play a role in the years ahead, eliminating the long wait for donors and the danger of tissue rejection. Physicians have used stem cell-derived tissues to treat patients with other disorders. But creating a functioning organ from stem cells is still a long way off.

Other possibilities include a bionic (human-made) face—an engineered prosthesis controlled by information coming from the brain—although such faces might not be natural-looking. Bionic hands are in development and may serve as a model for bionic faces. It may be possible in the future to make 3D-printed models of bones and other tissues now transplanted from donors, as well as 3D-printed cells.

The future of face transplants also depends on new attitudes from healthcare insurers. Andy's transplant was the first in the United States performed strictly under clinical protocols, not as a research procedure. The previously experimental character of the surgery made insurers unwilling to underwrite costs, and Andy's surgery was approved by Mayo as a charity case. But this is not a sustainable business model for transplant centers to follow.

What is needed, says Lori Ewoldt, Mayo's now-retired transplant administrator, is "a more evolved definition of lifesaving—you can leave the house again, you can eat food, you can smell, you can swim. Those are life's daily sustaining events, and they're also joyous events." And Ewoldt emphasizes that face transplants can save money over a series of reconstructive face surgeries.

When Mayo's transplant team compared the cost of a face transplant with the cost of the multiple stages and surgeries needed to continue with conventional reconstructive techniques, it found the path of a face transplant to be less costly while producing a better outcome for the patient. Mardini hopes that insurers will soon understand the unique role face transplants play in improving the function and quality of life of patients like Andy.

# Acknowledgments

———

This book would have remained unwritten without the help and cooperation of many people. I am grateful to Andy Sandness and the members of his family. They have allowed me to examine private events in their lives, some of them painful. Andy gave me access to his medical record as well.

For their participation and enthusiasm, I thank the dozens of Mayo Clinic staff members I interviewed, notably Samir Mardini, Hatem Amer, and Sheila Jowsey-Gregoire. I also thank Mayo photographers Eric Sheahan and Kevin Ness, who diligently recorded events with their cameras. I emerged from writing this book impressed by the commitment and skills of all the people I met who are involved in the care of patients at Mayo. In the same way, I salute the work of the people I interviewed at LifeSource. It's worth noting that this story began more than two decades ago. In some cases, people mentioned in the book may no longer be employed by Mayo or LifeSource.

This book would not exist without the spark, planning, and work of my partners at Mayo Clinic Press, including Daniel Harke, Nina Wiener, and Kelly Hahn. The work of editor Rachel Haring Bartony substantially improved the manuscript. Designer Amanda Knapp skillfully put it all together to create the book you hold in your hands.

My editor Philip Turner has been an energetic supporter from the very beginning. He took what was rough and made it smooth. My literary agent, Laura Langlie, gave her customary guidance. As always, my wife, Ann Aronson, served as my personal sounding board and voice of reason.

# Glossary

———

**Anaplastology.** A branch of medicine that blends art and science to create highly realistic prosthetic parts customized to fit individual specifications.

**Biopsy.** A procedure to remove a sample of tissue for testing in a laboratory.

**Brain death.** The donor's brain functions, including those of the brain stem, have ceased. Respiration, blood circulation, and other essential functions can be mechanically maintained if needed.

**Cadaver lab.** A specialized area containing cadavers that have been donated for the purpose of advancing medicine and science. Medical professionals come to learn essential parts of anatomy and surgery. Cadaver sessions are reputed to be the best available substitute for live surgery. They allow surgical trainees as well as experienced surgeons to gain a direct understanding and perspective of surgical anatomy. Surgeons develop anatomical awareness of different structures and manipulation of these structures.

**Craniofacial surgery.** A surgical specialty within the medical field of plastic surgery that treats and reconstructs disfigurements of the face, skull, and jaws.

**Cytomegalovirus.** A virus that a large portion of the population is exposed to. It may be carried in an inactive state for life by healthy individuals. It is a cause of severe pneumonia in people with a suppressed immune system, such as those undergoing bone marrow transplantation, those with leukemia or lymphoma, or those on immunosuppression therapy following organ transplantation. The acronym used for this virus is CMV.

**Dermatopathology.** A branch of medicine that studies diseases of the skin. A dermatopathologist examines tissue specimens under a microscope to make a diagnosis.

**Epstein-Barr virus (EBV).** A common virus that remains dormant in most people. EBV causes infectious mononucleosis and has been associated with certain cancers. In immuno-compromised people, this virus can cause abnormal production of white blood cells called lymphocytes. This can lead to lymphoproliferative diseases, including blood cancers.

**Exposure therapy.** In this form of therapy, psychologists create a safe environment in which to "expose" individuals to the things they fear and avoid. The exposure to the feared objects, activities, or situations in a safe environment helps reduce fear and decrease avoidance.

**Flap.** A section of tissue with its own blood supply taken from one area of the body and relocated to another to reconstruct an area damaged by injury or disease. Flaps are the best approach for covering large defects or when complex tissue is required to regain normal appearance. Examples include taking abdominal fat to reconstruct a breast or taking a portion of the fibula (a leg bone) and molding it to create a jawbone. The blood vessels in the transplanted tissue are connected to blood vessels in the reconstructed area so that the grafted tissue maintains healthy blood flow.

**Gastrostomy.** Insertion of a tube through the abdomen and into the stomach. The tube, also called a feeding tube, delivers liquid nutrition directly to the stomach. It's used when a person is unable to eat through their mouth for an extended period.

**Histocompatibility.** The degree of similarity between the genes of two individuals that helps predict how well a transplant recipient will tolerate a donor's tissue.

**Immunosuppression.** Suppression of the body's immune system and its ability to fight infections and other diseases. Immunosuppressant therapy is imperative after transplant surgery to minimize rejection of the new organ. Examples of immunosuppressant medications include prednisone, cyclosporine, mycophenolate mofetil, and tacrolimus.

**Informed consent.** A process by which a patient acquires relevant information from many sources and is educated with respect to his or her care, so that they can make decisions regarding proposed treatments based on a thorough understanding of all aspects of the procedures and care.

**Innervation.** The distribution or supply of nerves and nerve input to a body part.

**Invasive squamous cell carcinoma.** Squamous cell carcinoma is a common type of skin cancer that most often occurs on sun-exposed skin. When it grows beyond the layers of the skin and penetrates to deeper structures, it is referred to as invasive.

**Maxillofacial mandibular plating systems.** Systems of metal plates and screws, usually made of titanium, used to support jaw reconstruction surgery.

**Oculoplastic surgery.** A surgical specialty that focuses on procedures involving the eye and surrounding structures, including the eyelids, eye sockets (orbits), and tear drainage system.

**Oral endotracheal tube.** A breathing tube placed through the mouth into the windpipe (trachea).

**Oral mucosa.** The soft tissue membrane that lines the inside of the mouth. The oral mucosa is sensitive to touch and taste, but also acts as a protective barrier and produces substances to keep the mouth moist.

**Orbital floor.** Thin facial bones that provide support for the eyeballs.

**Pedicle.** A narrow strip of tissue, which includes an artery and a vein, linking the original site of a tissue graft to the transplant site. The pedicle provides a blood supply to the grafted tissue.

**Piezoelectric saw.** A cutting tool that uses ultrasonic vibrations to cut through bone. It's an alternative to mechanical and electrical instruments that lessens the risk of damage to surrounding soft tissue.

**Rejection.** An immune system response identifying transplanted tissue as foreign, triggering a cascade of biological events that may ultimately destroy the transplanted organ or tissue. Long-term survival of the transplant can be maintained by manipulating the immune system with immunosuppressant therapy to reduce the risk of rejection. Mild rejection episodes can often be managed with medication.

**Reconstructive microsurgery.** A surgical specialty that focuses on reconstructing any damaged part of the body. The field relies on understanding the blood supply and functions of different parts of the body. Body parts—often noses, jaws, fingers, or toes, but really any part—can be molded and transplanted to create form and function. A reconstructive microsurgeon uses a powerful microscope to magnify a minute surgical area, and precision tools and stitches to connect delicate structures such as blood vessels and nerves.

**Rhinoplasty.** A surgery that shapes or reconstructs the nose.

**Sentinel flap.** A piece of the donor's skin that is grafted onto the transplant recipient, usually in the groin area. It serves as a frontline indicator of rejection. If the sentinel flap shows signs of rejection, the main transplant may be in danger of rejection, as well. In the case of face transplant, the sentinel flap also can be used for routine biopsies and questions of rejection, so that the face does not develop multiple scars over time.

**Surgical technologist.** A healthcare professional who assists surgeons, nurses, and other members of a surgical team during an operation. Duties may include setting up a sterile operating room, preparing the patient, passing instruments and supplies during surgery, and making sure instruments and supplies are all accounted for.

**Synkinesis.** Involuntary movement of a facial muscle caused by the voluntary contraction of another facial muscle, such as the eye moving upward when blinking. It is essentially a co-contraction of muscles.

**Telecanthus.** An increased distance between the inner corners of the eyelids.

**Tissue engineering.** The practice of combining living scaffolds, cells, and other biologically active molecules into functional tissues. The goal of tissue engineering is to assemble functional constructs that restore or improve damaged tissues or whole organs.

**Tissue expander.** A silicone balloon that is inserted under the skin and gradually filled with saline to stretch and expand the skin over time.

**Tolerance induction.** Enhancing a transplant recipient's tolerance for cells from another body.

**Tracheostomy.** An opening that surgeons make through the front of the neck and into the windpipe (trachea). A tube is placed into the opening to provide for the passage of air in and out. A tracheostomy helps a person breathe when the usual route is blocked or impaired.

**Vascularized composite allotransplantation (VCA).** The transplantation of multiple tissues including muscle, bone, nerve, and skin as a functional unit—such as a hand or face—from a deceased donor to a recipient with a severe injury.

**Ventilator.** A machine that pumps air into a person's airways to help the person breathe or breathes for them.

# Resources

———

This book includes accounts of suicide and attempted suicide. If you or someone you know struggles with suicidal thoughts or is in crisis, call or text 988 day or night to reach the Suicide and Crisis Lifeline. Or text HOME to 741741 anytime to contact a trained crisis counselor.

An abundance of resources exists for prospective organ donors and transplant recipients.

**Donate Life America** (https://donatelife.net) is an alliance of transplant organizations across the United States advocating for increased organ and tissue donations.

**LifeSource** (www.life-source.org), active in many areas of the transplant and organ donation process in its region of the Upper Midwest, helps donors, patients, and their families.

**New England Donor Services** (https://neds.org/) coordinates organ and tissue donation in the New England area. It has also helped donor families involved in face transplants.

**The U.S. Health Resources & Services Administration** (www.organdonor.gov) has additional information on organ donation and instructions on how to sign up to be an organ donor.

**Transplant Living** (https://transplantliving.org) focuses on patients and their needs before and after their surgeries. Their website also hosts listings of local support groups by state for transplant patients and their families.

**The Organ Procurement and Transplantation Network** (https://optn.transplant.hrsa.gov) is a partnership between public and private institutions. It oversees the national organ transplant system. The network links all medical professionals involved in transplant in the U.S. It has a board of directors and committees that develop and oversee rules and policies governing the transplant system.

**The United Network for Organ Sharing** (www.unos.org) is a nonprofit scientific and educational organization that currently holds the contract granted by the OPTN. UNOS uses a computer system to match recipients and donors in an equitable way. It follows policies developed by the OPTN. The system continuously looks for matches to maximize the chances of successful transplantation.

# Selected Sources

———

In addition to interviews and medical records, secondary sources contributed much to the research for this book. Here is a partial list of the articles, books, and other published works that provided valuable background information.

Alberti, Fay Bound, and Victoria Hoyle. "Face Transplants: An International History." *Journal of the History of Medicine and Allied Sciences* 76, no. 3 (September 2021).

Austin, Jennifer. "Mayo Clinic's First Facial Transplant Recipient Speaks About Mental Health." KARE 11, September 26, 2019. https://www.kare11.com/article/news/local/mayo -clinic-face-transplant-recipient-shares-story/89-619e90dd-3f18 -49db-bf61-d6d0a5e33b7f.

Bever, Lindsey. "The Unforgettable Moment a Widow Touched the Face That Once Belonged to Her Husband." *Denver Post,* November 10, 2017.

Biernoff, Suzannah. "Theatres of Surgery: The Cultural Pre-History of the Face Transplant." Wellcome Open Research, May 8, 2018. https://wellcomeopenresearch.org/articles/3-54/v1.

Bowerman, Mary. "Woman Who Received World's First Face Transplant Dies." *USA Today,* September 7, 2016.

Bramstedt, Katrina A. "A Lifesaving View of Vascularized Composite Allotransplantation: Patient Experience of Social Death Before and After Face, Hand, and Larynx Transplant." *Journal of Patient Experience* 5, no. 2 (October 6, 2017).

Bromwich, Jonah Engel. "Isabelle Dinoire Dies at 49; Received First Partial Face Transplant Operation." *New York Times,* September 18, 2016.

Cohen, Sharon. "Face Transplant Patient's Hope After Twin Tragedies." Associated Press, February 18, 2017. https://www.news.com.au/lifestyle/real-life/true-stories/new-hope-for-face-transplant-patient-after-twin-tragedies/news-story/304f08257c6773c7ae1e983ae15c1c6e.

Concar, David. "The Boldest Cut." *New Scientist,* May 29, 2004.

Connors, Joanna. "Katie's New Face." *National Geographic,* September 2018.

"Face Transplant Recipient's Donor Face Now Failing."
Associated Press, September 22, 2019. https://apnews.com/2c39
d6ffa8c6466f884b19d6050db376.

Garrel-Jaffrelot, Tanguy. "Frenchman Who Got Face Transplant
in 2010 Is the First to Receive a Second." *New York Times,* April
20, 2018.

Goffman, Erving. *The Presentation of Self in Everyday Life.* New
York: Anchor, 1959.

Jowsey-Gregoire, Sheila, and Martin Kumnig. "Standardizing
Psychosocial Assessment for Vascularized Composite
Allotransplantation." *Current Opinion in Organ Transplantation*
21, no. 5 (October 2016).

Khatchadourian, Raffi. "How Dallas Wiens Found a New Face."
*The New Yorker,* February 5, 2012.

Kimberly, Laura L., Allyson R. Alfonso, Elie P. Ramly, Rami S.
Kantar, Arthur L. Caplan, and Eduardo D. Rodriguez. "How to
Integrate Lived Experience into Quality-of-Life Assessment in
Patients Considering Facial Transplantation." *AMA Journal of
Ethics,* November 2019.

Lamm, Bri. "Two Men Attempt Suicide Ten Years Apart—Only
One Succeeded." FaithIt, February 17, 2017. https://faithit.com
/andy-sandness-facial-transplant-miracle/.

Leone, Beret. "Man Inspires Others Struggling with Mental
Health After Face Transplant." KTTC, September 26, 2019.
https://kttc.com/2019/09/26/man-inspires-others-struggling
-with-mental-health-after-face-transplant/.

Neibergall, Charlie. "Tearful Meeting for Pair Forever Linked by Face Transplant." KAAL-TV, November 10, 2017. https://www.kaaltv.com/news/transform-conference-mayo-clinic-face-transplant-andy-sandness-first-latest-rochester-mn/5507508/.

Pietsch, Bryan. "Connie Culp, First Face Transplant Recipient in U.S., Dies at 57." *New York Times,* August 1, 2020.

Potter, Kyle. "Widow Meets Man Who Received Husband's Face in Transplant." *Chicago Tribune,* November 10, 2017.

Razonable, Raymund, and Hatem Amer. "Application of a New Paradigm for Cytomegalovirus Disease Prevention in Mayo Clinic's First Face Transplant." Mayo Clinic Proceedings 94, no. 1 (2019).

Rifkin, William J., Rami S. Kantar, Safi Ali-Khan, Natalie M. Plana, J. Rodrigo Diaz-Siso, Manos Tsakris, and Eduardo D. Rodriguez. "Facial Disfigurement and Identity: A Review of the Literature and Implications for Facial Transplantation." *AMA Journal of Ethics,* April 2018.

Roth, Ian. "Two Years After Face Transplant, Andy's Smile Shows His Progress." Mayo Clinic, February 28, 2019. https://newsnetwork.mayoclinic.org/discussion/2-years-after-face-transplant-andy-sandness-smile-shows-his-progress/.

Scott, Paul. "Andy Sandness, First Mayo Face-Transplant, Tells Story of Pain and Renewal." *Rochester (MN) Post Bulletin,* September 27, 2019. https://www.postbulletin.com/lifestyle/andy-sandness-first-mayo-face-transplant-tells-story-of-pain-and-renewal.

Siemionow, Maria. "The Decade of Face Transplant Outcomes." *Journal of Materials Science: Materials in Medicine* 28, art. 64 (2017).

Starzl, Thomas E., and Clyde Barker. "The Shared Trail of Organ, Limb, and Face Transplantation." *Proceedings of the American Philosophical Society* 155, no. 1 (March 2011).

Staveley-Wadham, Rose. "A Gift of Warfare: The History of Plastic Surgery." *The British Newspaper Archive Blog,* January 21, 2021. https://blog.britishnewspaperarchive.co.uk/2021/01/21 /history-of-plastic-surgery.

Streed, Joel. "Andy's Smile Shows His Progress Two Years After Face Transplant." Mayo Clinic, March 29, 2019. https://sharing .mayoclinic.org/2019/03/29/andys-smile-shows-his-progress-two -years-after-face-transplant/.

Tiede, Hannah. "Face Transplant Recipient Transforming Lives with a Message of Hope." KAAL-TV, September 26, 2019. https://www.kaaltv.com/news/transform-conference-mayo -clinic-face-transplant-andy-sandness-first-latest-rochester -mn/5507508/.

# Index

## About Mayo Clinic and Mayo Clinic Transplant Center

Mayo Clinic is a nonprofit organization committed to innovation in clinical practice, education, and research and to providing compassion, expertise, and answers to everyone who needs healing.

Mayo Clinic Transplant Center performs more transplants at its Arizona, Florida, and Minnesota campuses combined than any other medical center in the nation. The integrated teams of surgeons, doctors, nurses, pharmacists, social workers, and others work together to manage every aspect of a patient's transplant, from planning of transplant options through post-transplant care.

Mayo Clinic Transplant Center's reconstructive transplant program is one of a few in the world that offers face and hand transplants as part of its clinical care. The program provides patients with facial and upper extremity deformities with the appropriate surgical procedure, from simple reconstruction to a face or hand transplant. Mayo Clinic performed its first face transplant in 2016 and its second in February 2024. The reconstructive transplant program's multidisciplinary team excels in complex operations and procedures to restore form and function to the face. The team's collective expertise has transformed lives, enabling patients to regain vital functions and improve quality of life.

Information on organ donation, tissue rejection, and conditions treatable by transplant can be found on the Transplant Center's website (www.mayoclinic.org/departments-centers/transplant-center). Look for the upcoming *Mayo Clinic Guide to Organ Transplant: The Comprehensive Guide for Patients from the World's Leading Transplant Experts*, to be published in 2026 by Mayo Clinic Press.

Scan to learn more about Andy Sandness
and the transformation of medicine